Towards a Theology of

HEALTHCARE

IN CREATION

James Thwaites

Teleios Resource Publishing

If transformation in healthcare for the glory of God is something you want to be involved in, you need to read James Thwaites' latest book. He will challenge your presuppositions and force you to re-think your world-view. This book will assist Christians to engage in a vigorous and in-depth conversation about the nature of God's purpose for healthcare and healing. I believe that this kind of enquiry and dialogue is exactly what is needed at this time.

Chris Steyn
International Coordinator
Healthcare Christian Fellowship, Europe

I first met James Thwaites shortly after the publication of his first book, The Church Beyond the Congregation, in the mid-nineties. We invited James to have input into our leadership team, in regards to the changes that were taking place at that time. We found his advice invaluable and it enabled us to transition smoothly to a new way of operating as 'church'. We have moved from being a congregation with quite a traditional focus to one with a stronger focus on encouraging and equipping people to fulfill their God-given destiny in every part of life.

In this transition, we have had to engage the Scriptures with a view to developing and/or revisiting theologies that apply to people's work in education, charities, government, healthcare and more. By way of example, a group of healthcare professionals have set up New Community Health in Southampton to provide health services across the city.

James' book, Towards a Theology of Healthcare in Creation, is a prime example of the kind of theological enquiry we need at this time. Speaking with James and having read much of the manuscript, I believe that this book will not only equip Christians in healthcare, but will also bring value and insight to many other spheres of work. I highly recommend this book to you.

Billy Kennedy leads the UK Pioneer with his wife Caroline.
He is also senior leader of New Community, Southampton,
a network of Christ-centered communities

Over the years I have been greatly influenced in my understanding of the biblical world-view by the teaching of James Thwaites. He provides an understanding of the huge influence of Plato and Aristotle on Western, scientific and medical thought and contrasts that with an Hebraic and biblical world-view, which is much more aligned to a holistic understanding of healthcare and healing.

His concept of the 'remedial space' is extremely helpful in working with people with a great range of illnesses and complex issues. His teaching and explorations in these areas are now produced in this book. I commend this book to all who practice in healthcare and those who are seeking a more biblical understanding of healthcare, illness, healing and wholeness.

Dr Ken Curry
Health Care in Christ, Australia

James Thwaites, in his latest book, Towards a Theology of Healthcare in Creation, invites us, as healthcare workers, into a space that may at first sight seem unfamiliar. Yet, as our vision becomes clearer, we begin to recognise it as a place we know well. This is the space of the healing room, where the healthcare worker and the sick person meet and address diagnosis and treatment, both in the conventional sense and in terms of the deeper meaning of the person's story in God.

James explores the concept of creation as being one vast 'remedial space' designed to bring people into more of life and health and maturity. In this, he does not tell us what we should or should not do. Rather, he opens up perspectives and insights from the Scriptures that enable us to engage in our work in healthcare in a renewed light. I have applied this 'remedial space' template to my work in pain management, and as a result have been able to make significant changes to my practice. I encourage you to explore more of this healing room of creation and thereby discover more of who you are in your work in healthcare.

Dr Chris Hayes
Pain Management Specialist,
Newcastle, Australia

Copyright © 2013 James Thwaites
Publisher: teleios resource: Sydney, Australia
email address: teleios_co@bigpond.com

PUBLISHING

www.teleios.org.au   FOLLOW US ON facebook

Paperback ISBN 978-0-9871706-2-0

Printed in Australia, United Kingdom and the United States of America.
Distributed internationally by Ingram Book Group.

Available as an eBook through Amazon Kindle, Apple iBookstore and all major outlets.
eBook ISBN 978-0-9871706-1-3

The right of James Thwaites to be identified as the Author of this Work has been asserted by
him in accordance with the Copyright, Designs and Patents Act 1988. Unless otherwise stated,
Scripture quotations are taken from the New American Standard Bible ©.

Cover Design
J. Elliot, Graphic Design & Hannah Haynes, Art Therapist
Copy Editor: David Thwaites

CONTENTS

This book is dedicated to my father
Cedric F. Thwaites MB BS FRACS
Physician and Surgeon

Introduction to the Author

James Thwaites has written a number of books, variously described as exciting, clarifying and comprehensive. Those who know him personally see him as a down to earth and funny guy with an infectious passion for the church. James' insights have inspired many Christians around the world.

For 22 years James was an ordained minister of religion in Manly, Sydney, Australia. During this time he was involved in a number of community initiatives, including the establishment of a multi-disciplinary healthcare practice. In 1999, after 'blending' his congregation with another church congregation, James became an elder of the joint congregation.

The impact of his involvement in community initiatives caused James to reconsider the nature and role of the church, which resulted in the publication of three books. These books explored the church from the standpoint of the Hebraic world-view (as presented in Scripture), in contrast to what James believed was the historical influence of the Platonic (dualistic) world-view on our understanding of church. Published in the United Kingdom, the books are: *The Church Beyond the Congregation* (Paternoster, 1999); *Church that Works*, co-authored with David Oliver (Word Publishing, 2001); and *Renegotiating the Church Contract* (Paternoster, 2002).

The success of these publications has led James into speaking at conferences in many parts of the world. Given Jim's passion for seeing Christians more effective in their everyday work, it is no surprise that over time he was asked to bring his insights more directly into workplace settings. This led him to engage with many leaders in various spheres of work. He has since been engaged as a consultant in organisational leadership development, with a particular focus on ethical leadership.

James remains an elder in his local church and works with its leadership team. This team includes David Gore, the presiding minister. James lives in Sydney with his wife Margaret and their four children. This book is the fruit of many years of reflection and enquiry into the Scriptures. It has been tested and tried in many healthcare settings, in numerous conversations and many conferences. Not surprisingly, it has been long awaited by many. I believe this book will prove to be a valuable and lasting resource for those who work in healthcare and believe the Judaeo-Christian Scriptures.

Stephen Baxter – friend and colleague,
Church Leader, Tasmania, Australia

Author's Preface

In early 1994 I established a multi-disciplinary healthcare practice, which included psychologists, doctors, counsellors, prayer teams and support groups. The team was made up of Christians who sought to apply their faith to their work in healthcare. It was a fruitful initiative that impacted for the good on both clients and practitioners. That being said, however, a few years into the practice it became evident to me that we had not been able to gain much theological ground. I knew, of course, that there was much divine wisdom in the Scriptures that we could apply to our work, but it seemed to me that we were not quite getting hold of it.

Once I became aware of this I started looking for answers. During our team meetings I began to notice that there were two well-defined language sets being used. The first expressed the teams religious/spiritual culture derived from their church theology, and the second was derived from the secular/material dimension of their profession and its practices and protocols. In our discussions both, of course, were valid; but the more I saw this language dynamic in action the more I realised that there was very little shared-space between the two. This insight helped me to understand the difficulty we faced in our endeavour to integrate the truths of Scripture with the practice of healthcare and healing.

As a minister of a church for twenty-three years, I had been aware of the impact of Plato's dualism on Christian thinking. I had also known for many years about the ancient Hebrew vision of God's creation (as believed by the prophets, apostles and Christ himself); but now I began to further enquire into these two different versions of seeing or understanding the universe. This led me to write my first book, *The Church Beyond the Congregation*. In that book I applied these two cosmologies (ie versions of the universe) to our understanding of the Fall. I will, of course, expand on these two approaches to creation reality in this book.

My conviction was (and still is) that Plato's cosmology influenced the early and mostly Gentile church to apply a frame of divine justice and punishment to most all that happened at the time of the Fall. The ancient Hebrews, on the other hand, were focused more on God's creation. As such, I believe their understanding of the Fall was seen in a different light to Christendom's long-held account of the Fall. And why, pray tell, would this have any bearing on one's practice of healthcare and healing?

In a book about a theology of healthcare in creation, it would stand to reason that an event, which is said by Christians to have generated all human pain, disease, decay and death, should be explored in the light of the ancient Hebrew vision of creation. This enquiry into Hebraic cosmology is not just about the Fall; it is about *'all creation under heaven'* (Col. 1:23). The key dividend of this exploration is what I describe as the remedial space design of creation. This divine design, encompassing God's creation, is akin to a vast healing room of life; designed, I believe, so that humans might choose life and maturity in God.

This remedial space design has been embraced by many healthcare practitioners as a means by which they can more fully understand and engage the divine nature and purpose of their work in healthcare and healing. This is the intent of this book; that Christians might establish stronger links between their work in healthcare and God's ultimate purpose for healthcare and healing.

Also to say, every person in some way or other will engage with pain, disease, decay and, ultimately, death. And most every person will in some way seek to understand the nature and/or meaning of these creation forces. As such, many of the issues and considerations we will explore throughout this book will not only be applicable to Christians working in healthcare, but also it will apply to everyday life.

A few house-keeping considerations are in order. In this book I use 'practitioner' and 'healthcare worker' to refer to medical, nursing and ancillary healthcare practitioners and psychological counsellors and/or therapists. Sometimes I will refer to 'we' or 'us' when referring to this group, as I am also involved in counselling and therapeutic work.

Throughout the book I will use phrases such as 'healthcare practitioners who believe'. At other times I simply refer to healthcare practitioners or healthcare workers without referencing the word 'believer' or 'follower of Christ'; this because it would encumber the text to do otherwise. Also, it might help readers of other religious persuasions to have more affinity with the book.

Most of the Scriptural references in the book are drawn from the New American Standard Bible (NASB). I also draw from Alfred Marshall's NASB Interlinear Greek-English New Testament (Regency. US. 1984). At times, I will replace part of an NASB text with wording from the interlinear translation, so as to emphasise certain points. I tag these 'hybrid' verses with the abbreviation 'ILGE'. All added emphases are mine. Finally, do bear in mind that when it comes to seeing the ancient Hebrew vision of life in God, it is more important at first to get the picture than it is to get the point.

James Thwaites. 2013.
Sydney, Australia

01

Healthcare, Creation and Cosmology

In my experience over many years in conversations with healthcare workers who are Christian, I have often noted the division that exists between their faith and their work. Yes, the connection is there when it comes to their being responsible, honest, caring and prayerful. When I ask healthcare workers to speak about how they apply the Scriptures to their everyday work in healthcare, the qualities I referred to are often mentioned. If I push a bit further and ask them about their theological understanding of healthcare practice, most don't quite know how to respond to the question itself. I then prompt them, by way of references to the Fall, and they do begin to talk about God's curse and how death and disease were introduced as punishments for sin. My next question to them is: 'does any of this theology of the Fall impact on their everyday healthcare practice?' In reply, some say 'I suppose so'; but most say something like 'no, it doesn't really impact on what I do in my everyday work'.

When it comes to spheres of work, such a business or government or media, the Fall would not be something that would often weigh on the minds of Christians in those workplaces. But when it comes to healthcare, with its focus on disease, suffering, decay and death – all of which are said to exist because of the Fall – it should be the case that Christians in healthcare would have a greater awareness of the relationship between their work and the effects of the Fall. To put it another way: is it not strange that two-thousand years and more after the coming of God the Son made man, of whom Paul said, *'by him all things were created, both in the heavens and on earth, visible and invisible'* (Col. 1:16), that there exists such a frail and confused connection between Christian theology and healthcare practice?

My intent in this book is to expand and strengthen our understanding of these connections; this so that Christians in healthcare and healing professions might gain more insight into the nature and divine purpose of their work. I hasten to add at this point that I will not be advocating for some new form of Bible-based medical practice – perish the thought! Rather, I am focused, as was Paul the apostle, on *'equipping... the saints for the work of service'* (Eph. 4:12). This *'equipping'* will not involve me directly in commentary on medical/healthcare practices. Rather, my focus is on the creation; it being the key context within which, I believe, the above-stated intent will be realised.

cosmological options

It goes without saying, but it needs to be said: for those who believe in Christ, it is essential that their vision of the universe aligns with the one who created it. For those brought up in a Western European culture there are three main versions of the universe on offer. The first comes from the Greek philosopher Plato (427-347BC), the second arises from a mix of Aristotle (384-322BC) and Copernicus (1473-1543AD) and the third is the Hebraic vision of creation, as depicted in the Judeo-Christian Scriptures. At this stage in history, the dominant cosmology of Western civilisation is that which derives from the philosophy of Aristotle and Copernicus.

Definition of cosmology: 1. the philosophical study of the origin and nature of the universe. 2. The branch of astronomy concerned with the evolution and structure of the universe. *Collins English Dictionary* (Wm. Collins Publishers, reprint 1980).

When it comes to Christians, it would stand to reason that they would put their hands up for the Hebrew version of the universe. Not so. The reason for this is that very early in the history of the church, circa third century AD, the mostly Gentile church put their hands up for Plato's version of reality. Such was the influence of Plato's cosmology that he was (almost) given a posthumous seat in the Roman Church. Jonathon Sachs, the recently retired Chief Rabbi of the Commonwealth, says of Plato that *'Alfred North Whitehead once said that Western philosophy was "a series of footnotes to Plato". He might have put it more strongly: Not just philosophy but Western religion has been haunted by Plato's ghost'. The Dignity of Difference* (Continuum, 2002), p. 20.

This begs the question: to what extent has Plato influenced Christianity's understanding of the Fall? Yes, it is a big question, particularly when it comes to us deciding what we believe about the nature and purpose of disease, suffering, decay and death. For my part, I believe that Adam and Eve sinned and God intervened via judgement; a judgement that has profoundly affected not only humanity but also the entire creation. Like many other teachers and ministers of religion, I have difficulty in making sense of God's radical response to the first couple's sin. I am aware that tampering with long-held doctrines, particularly the doctrine of the Fall, is a risky business. My conviction is, however, that what happened at the time of the Fall does need to be re-examined in the light of Plato's influence. In the following chapter I will begin my critique on Plato's version of the universe.

living by the fall

For now, let's turn to the standard historical version of what is said to have happened at time of the Fall and beyond. Adam and Eve sin, and in response, God radically changes the entire creation, introducing pain, disease, decay and death to all of humanity. This creation, which was once the means by which humanity would grow up and mature in God and his purpose (as per the Genesis 1:28 mandate), was now placed under a curse, and effectively pushed aside in God's plan for humans. Further to this, theologians tell us that this first sin caused every person who ever lived (minus Christ) to be born spiritually dead to God and sinful by nature. Some go even further, saying that, post-Fall, God gave the devil control over this cursed creation and its corrupted humanity.

It's quite a story, not one that you would read to your young children before they go to bed at night! Reading this unabashed version of the Fall, it's easy to see why Christians working in healthcare find it difficult to integrate their religious beliefs into their everyday practice. In effect, they have been told by church leaders and theologians that disease, suffering, decay and death are products of divine wrath and punishment. Hardly any Christian I know is able to consistently live in a world that is defined in this way. It is for this reason that most of them compromise by identifying their theology with religious ideas and church activities, and from there associating their working and personal life, for the most part, with the culture of the day.

My conviction is that this *split* between life and religion has beggared the church, diminishing its power and confusing its divine purpose. Hence my desire to revisit the doctrine of the Fall, via help from the ancient Hebrew vision of God's creation. My hope is that we might listen anew to what God said to Adam and Eve on that fateful and fallen day in Eden. I will begin this exploration into Eden in chapter three.

physical theology

One of the biggest challenges I will face in achieving my goal for this book will be to persuade readers to believe that the physical creation holds an essential key to God's plan for us humans. A part of this challenge is that Christendom's version of the Fall states that creation has been cursed by God and substantially written off in the divine plan. The idea that there would be an in-depth theology of the physical creation is simply not on our religious radar. By way of example, I have repeatedly asked a friend in Leeds UK – an academic focused on the mining industry – to supply me with a simple or basic theology of mining. He knows there is one there, but after several years he still cannot access it. It is of note, in this regard, that most every pronouncement made by God at the time of the Fall had to do with the physical realm, eg the increase of thorns and thistles, the curse in the ground, multiplied pain in childbirth and the physical death of the human body.

Paul, the Hebrew of Hebrews, said that *'the spiritual is not first, but the natural; then the spiritual'* (1 Cor. 15:46). He also said that *'since the creation of the world [God's] invisible attributes, his eternal power and divine nature, have been clearly seen, being understood through what has been made'* (Rom. 1:20). What is apparent to me in these verses is that if we do not engage the physical creation we will find it very difficult to properly engage the spiritual aspects of life.

earth – not the center

There are other hindrances in the way of understanding God's creation. One such obstacle arises from the church's retreat from cosmology into the relative safety of one's world-view. Note: the *Collins English Dictionary* describes world-view as *'a comprehensive view or personal philosophy of human life and the universe'*. This 'retreat' owes a good deal to the idea that creation, post-Fall, is said to be cursed and corrupted. But there is more; it having to do with a somewhat embarrassing church incident that happened towards the end of the middle ages.

Four centuries before Christ, the philosopher Aristotle came to believe that the earth was located at the center of the universe. Twelve centuries after Christ rose from the dead, the Roman Catholic church bought into Aristotle's idea; so much so that they made a doctrine of it. One day, however, Nicolaus Copernicus (as mentioned earlier on in this chapter) suggested that the earth was not the center of anything. Instead, he believed that the sun was the center of the universe.

This shift in cosmology did not initially raise any eyebrows on the part of the clerics. But once Copernicus published his book on the subject (and died soon afterwards) certain church leaders began to get nervous; they being accustomed to infallibility. Over time, both Catholics and Protestants began to take issue with this idea. By 1616AD it was one very hot topic; so much so that Galileo Galilei was directed by the Catholic Church to cease from speaking about this apparent heresy.

To make a long story short: in time it became obvious that the church had got it wrong. From that time on, the church, both Catholic and Protestant, has been for the most part deathly quiet when it comes to the issue of cosmology; it now preferring the softer touch of world-viewing. Of course, Copernicus' findings were also modified over time; in that the sun was also not the center of the universe. But again to say, it was he who started this cosmological revolution – thereby diminishing the status of the long-held Catholic doctrine of infallibility.

revisiting your cosmos

I encourage the reader to not be alarmed. I am not about to storm the citadels of science with some new news about an ancient Middle-Eastern cosmology. Also, I do not plan to discuss how long it took the infinite God to make the first second of space-time and matter. Yes, I have my own thoughts about monkeys and humans and their relationship to each other, but this is not my concern here. I do believe, however, that the church's theological retreat from cosmology has left far too much behind in its wake. I would go so far as to say that in our flight of embarrassed confusion we left most of God's good creation in the dust of our withdrawal; thereby handing over most of creation to those who engage and sum up reality via the measurements of matter, maths and physical laws.

As I indicated in the preface, this book is an enquiry into humanity's relationship to God and his creation, as viewed from the ancient Hebrew vision. My particular emphasis will be on creation forces such as pain, disease, decay and death and our human response to them, specifically from healthcare and healing practitioners. To achieve this goal we will, of course, need to search the Scriptures. This exploration will at times lead us into some unfamiliar theological territory. I can say, however, that in the past fourteen or so years I have tested my findings, both from the Scriptures and from many individuals working in healthcare. It is from this enquiry that the remedial space design of creation has emerged.

Of course, this creation design has been there all along, and, as such, each of us has experienced it in some way, shape or form. But again to say, it is the ancient Hebraic vision of heaven and earth that has brought this divine design into focus. This remedial space design will not and should not tell healthcare workers what to do by way of their day-to-day practice; rather, this creation design serves to establish a larger context within which they can progressively discover more of God's wisdom in their work in healthcare and healing. I call this context – 'God's creation sphere of healthcare and healing'.

book designs

I will sign off on this first chapter by giving a very brief overview of the book. Chapter two looks in more detail at Plato's impact on our understanding of the Fall. Chapters three to five give a detailed summary of Hebraic cosmology. From there, in chapters six to ten, I apply this Hebraic understanding to the physical forces that impact on the human body – and, thereby, on the human being. Chapters eleven and twelve focus on the remedial space design and its divine process and purpose.

Chapters thirteen and fourteen look into the application of this remedial space design to healthcare workers in everyday life. Also in these chapters I begin to look (in part) into what I believe is God's creation strategy for healthcare and healing. Chapters fourteen and fifteen continue this theological approach to divine strategy – of course, from an Hebraic standpoint. Chapter sixteen is hard to describe, so I will let the reader decide what it might mean to them!

Let's now proceed to Athens, 5th century BC, there to find out how one man divided and conquered the minds of so many, thereby significantly shutting down their vision of life in God's creation. This man's name? Plato.

02

Plato Takes Hold of the Universe

Plato was a philosopher and a genius. There is no doubting the depths of many of the insights he had into the human condition. That being said, there are two streams in any text. The first is the content and the second is the intent. The philosopher, Karl Popper, in his book *The Open Society and its Enemies, Vol. 1, The Spell of Plato* (London: Routledge, 1966, reprint 1989) asserts that Plato's intent in writing *The Republic* had most to do with his desire to win back the rule of Athens, which had been taken from him and his aristocratic clan by the Democrats.

The plan Plato employed was an old one; that being to first divide and then to conquer. What was unique about his strategy, however, was that the division he sought was not between peoples or groups, but rather it set-up shop in the mind of the individual. How did he do this? Plato began by saying that the material world around us was not true reality. Instead it was just a corrupted copy of the real and perfect realm that existed outside of the present creation. It was in this perfect realm that these 'eternal ideas' existed, of which the physical forms on earth were only a pale imitation.

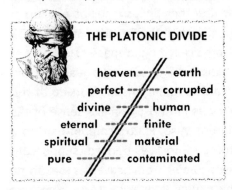

THE PLATONIC DIVIDE

heaven ---/--- earth
perfect ---/--- corrupted
divine ---/--- human
eternal ---/--- finite
spiritual ---/--- material
pure ---/--- contaminated

In effect, Plato established a belief in the mind of his followers that life was divided into two compartments, each containing a nature that is the opposite of the other. Why would a person do such a thing? Plato wanted to affect a profound sense of psychological deficit in people. This would arise in the mind of any person who came to believe that they lived in 'the wrong place' and needed to get out of there and into 'the right place'. Plato effectively created a 'dis-ease' in the human mind. His reason for doing this was to make people dependent on a cure that only he could supply. This cure was an entity called 'the State' – a ruling body whose nature and authority was established by turning those 'eternal ideas' that came from the eternal realm into laws. If a person came under the rule of Plato's State they would be eligible to align with the dictates and dogmas coming down from the eternal realm; thereby giving them a chance to get through to Plato's version of salvation. So it was that the long-standing saying about the divine right of kings to rule was changed to read 'the divine right of (selected) eternal ideas to rule'. From there Plato declared that his ruling 'idea-run' State should in turn be ruled by what he called a 'philosopher king'. Less than subtle, is it not? Is it any wonder that the Athenian Democrats said no?

Several centuries on, however, the early church said yes, and once the marriage was sealed, Plato's cosmology came into its own. By 500AD a church that God designed to be a body of people standing in Christ in every sphere of life in creation (as per Eph. 1:22-23) had become a whole lot like Plato's State – a power structure separated from everyday Christians, transformed into a mediating 'construct' between this life and the next. It was this form of church, under Caesar's patronage, that took charge of the religious part of the Roman Empire.

philosopher gets lucky

I would imagine that some readers at this stage might ask the question: why Plato and not, say, any number of philosophers and/or religions that were on offer in this era? The reason is that no other philosopher or religion at that time came close to being able to identify with the Christian story. Plato's take on creation as being a corrupted, physically-bound mass of chaos was considered to align with the curse and chaos that was said to have arisen from the Fall. Plato's vision of a far-removed divine realm existing outside of this sordid creation enabled the Gentile believers in Christ to make sense of the heaven of God they read about in Scripture. Also, Plato's commitment to a ruling State, established by concepts turned into laws derived, supposedly, from the eternal realm, was akin to Christ's coming from heaven as the 'divine logos' to establish the church. It was this church, fed fat by Rome, that gave birth to a mediating construct ruled over by theological kings whose job it was to manage the flow of believers between the finite creation and Plato's version of the eternal/heavenly realm.

Not only did Plato assist Christians in making sense of Christ, he also offered Christianity access to the predominately Greek culture of that era. In effect, the Platonic version of reality became an apologetic for Christianity. This marriage between Plato and the church has continued all the way through the Reformation period and beyond to this day.

When it came to Plato's influence on the church's understanding of the Fall, the first causality was the creation itself – it being essentially written off in-line with the philosopher's cosmology. From there, the natural realm became just a cursed and sordid back-drop to the spiritual action, which mostly took place between the mediating construct of the church and the supposed heavenly courts of divine justice.

IDEAS THAT COME TO RULE

The philosopher, Karl Popper, names Plato as the father of Western ideology. To this day the tendency for a chosen few to take charge of a body of knowledge, and then use that knowledge to take charge – be that in a nation (fascism, communism) or a discipline (economics, science), or a religion (Christianity, Islam) – is indeed strong. The process by which an ideology emerges is very simple. First you acquire an idea/truth and emphasise its importance over other related ideas/truths. From there you will need to convince people to follow you by believing in your idea/truth. This is more likely to happen if you tell them that your idea/truth is universal or divine in origin. Once your followers are in place, along with the infrastructure to support your ruling idea/truth, you will have completed the journey from idea to ideal to ideology – and then, to control.

---

impact statements

In the prior chapter I referred to the difficulty Christians have in making sense of the Fall in their everyday life; particularly those who work in healthcare and healing professions. I will now add several 'impact statements' from a person who has tried very hard to combine their understanding of the Fall with their work as a doctor of medicine. Her name is Meredith Long. She wrote a book titled *Health, Healing and God's Kingdom – New Pathways to Christian Health Ministry in Africa*, (Regnum, UK, 2000). The book is insightful and informative, particularly in regards to how the indigenous African experience of life in creation contrasts with the Western and Christian approach to healthcare and healing. What stands out to me, however, is the challenge Long has when it comes to interpreting her research through the theological framework she has been taught. Speaking of God's judgements at the time of the Fall (the curse, as she calls it) Long's challenge, to my mind, becomes evident – as per the following quote from her book.

'Despite the effects of the curse, men and women throughout the world cultivate the land, tend their flocks and harness the latent energy of creation to survive and often to prosper. Medical science is itself an exploration in dominion. The work of development agencies in _countering the effects of God's curse_ in enabling men and women to exercise creative dominion over the environment is part of the redemptive work of God, _even though its impact is temporary_' (p. 44).

Of course, on one level I can understand what is being said here, in that God's judgements at the Fall do not require of us that we multiply their adverse effects by our actions. Rather, we should try to mitigate them. My issue is not so much with lessening the impact of God's judgement. What I am focusing on is a perception on the part of Long that she is engaged in a work on behalf of a good God that works against God's own intention to judge and to punish people for Adam's sin.

To me this is akin to a kingdom with divided intents – working for an outcome whilst working against it. As Jesus said in relation to such a setup, a Kingdom divided cannot stand; the reason being that it lives in contradiction and thereby works against itself. As a sad sign off to her words, Long says that at the end of all her work, she will not succeed in overcoming God's curse. All her efforts and their impacts are just temporary measures that will ultimately give way to the forces of wrath, decay and death. This is the story she has been told by her church. This is the story she has to keep trying to live and work with.

misplaced God

Long, like others, cannot stay in a zone in which God is seen to be against her work, whilst at the same time being in support of her work, with God's hand against life winning out in the end. To help her cope, she has to blur the image of the God of wrath and punishment on her canvass of life and paint it over with the shapes and colours of an inanimate, capricious and quasi-divine force called 'nature' – as per her following statements:

'The natural forces designed by God to express the goodness of his creation are the same ones that work towards its destruction.' *'Creation is the source of wealth and beauty, but it is also a terrible enemy.'* *'As part of the curse, work as creative stewardship has been compromised and become, in part, a battle for survival.'* *'In God's judgement of sin the wilderness of creation is transformed to hostility.'* (p. 43). The above quotes suggest to me that many Christians, including Long, seem to be regularly experiencing a form of 'God disassociation'. In one instance God is active in cursing and judging the creation, but then suddenly in our minds this same God goes missing from creation, with inanimate forces taking up the cudgel and whip on behalf of the now (apparently) absented divine. It is these kinds of statements from a Christian working in the hard places of life that cause me to think that Plato has been a greater influence on Christian theology than Christ himself.

a cosmological option

I am not saying that the theologians and church leaders who have influenced Long have their doctrines entirely wrong. My challenge is that many of these doctrines have been placed in a cosmological framework that owes much to Plato's dualism. So many Christians, including Long, have tried very hard for so long to work with the current church account of the Fall, but still they find themselves unable to make sense of its divided story. If there was no other account, no other way of understanding what happened to humanity and creation at the Fall, then so be it. But what if there was another option drawn from the Scriptures? Surely we would want to examine it and see how it might fit with the Genesis chapter 3 narrative. There is such a one; that being the Hebraic vision of *'all creation under [God's] heaven'* (Col. 1:23). Surely, we must not overlook such an vision as this.

Let's now see how well the Hebraic cosmology fits with the standard account of the Fall. To do this we will at first need to ask the ruling idea of 'divine justice as punishment for sin' to take a seat, but not a ruling seat; and yes, to be present, but no longer taking charge of proceedings. With this polite protocol in place, we now proceed to Eden.

03

Intervention
in the Garden

As much as most theologians think that the Genesis 3 mandate for humanity was withdrawn at the time of the Fall, I beg to differ. All one needs to do is to read Psalm 8, written in the post-Fall period, and see that our creation mandate to steward, subdue and thereby ultimately come *'to rule over the works of [God's] hands'* (Ps. 8:6) is still very much in play. Once we are in tune with this information, and are willing to get going to *'fill the earth'* (Gen. 1:28), we can begin to make lots more connections to the present creation.

The truth is that from the beginning God made creation for humans and humans for creation. Yes, it's true – they are made for each other. I call this a 'counterpart relationship' in which when one party changes the other party responds accordingly. *Collins English Dictionary* describes 'counterpart' as *'one of two parts that complement or correspond to each other'*. This dynamic is well in evidence in the pre-Fall Genesis account. When Adam and Eve were created in innocence the creation was wild and needing to be tamed. It was that untamed state that indicated to them their need of growth and maturity. As they related to the creation, drawing wisdom and resources from that engagement, they would have grown up in relationship to creation, and to God, and thereby in time come to inherit, firstly the earth and then the human and angelic heavens over that earth – as per Hebrews 2:7. Again to say, it would have been the progressively changing state of the creation, from sea to land to sky, that would have indicated and thus reflected back to humans how far they had come in fulfilling God's purpose.

If creation has been made by God so that you and I could grow and mature in our relationship to him, would it not be strange that God would judge Adam and Eve by re-designing the creation in such a way that the life-connections between them would be severed, with the creation now becoming their enemy? A good judge is one who intervenes in such a way that the reality or consequences of a person's actions might be known and appropriately dealt with. As such, would it not be consistent for God, post-Fall, to have changed creation in such a way that it would be able to continually relate to humans in their fallen state? Wouldn't it make sense

> 'It is [God] who made the earth by his power, who established the world by his wisdom; and by his understanding he has stretched out the heavens'
> Jeremiah 10:12

that when humanity 'fell' that the creation would shift and change to match that 'fall'? With that in view let's look again at God's pronouncements at the Fall and from this 'creation-as-counterpart' perspective gain a sense of the spirit and intent of his words in response to the sin of Adam and Eve.

the ground judges?

God's says to Adam: *'Because you have listened to the voice of your wife, and have eaten from the tree about which I commanded you, saying, 'You shall not eat from it': Cursed is the ground because of you; In toil you shall eat of it all the days of your life. Both thorns and thistles it shall grow for you; And you shall eat the plants of the field; By the sweat of your face you shall eat bread till you return to the ground, because from it you were taken; For you are dust, and to dust you shall return'* (Gen. 3:17-19).

The first thing to note in this passage is that God's judgement is not directly given to Adam; instead it arises from the ground – as in *'cursed is the ground because of you'*. Of course, Adam is very much in view here, but the focus of this judgement and its consequences is on the ground of earth. It is a fascinating turn of phrase God employs here. The ground is cursed, not because of the demands of divine justice or wrath; rather, it is cursed *'because of you'* Adam. In line with the 'creation-as-counterpart' dynamic, it is the ground that makes evident the consequences of Adam's actions.

Of course, God is most certainly the first cause of this consequence of sin; as it is God who has designed and made the ground that is now responding to Adam in this way. God is most definitely in this action, both as its initial designer and as the one delivering the news of what now will happen to Adam and Eve. As such, one need not fear that creation is engaging in some kind of independent activity 'other' to God. It is not. God has made creation to work in line with his divine nature and eternal purpose. As our counterpart, the creation is simply doing what it is designed to do, which is to respond by continuing to match the new-found state of post-Fall humanity.

the divine commentary

God continues, saying to Adam in relation to this curse from the ground that now *'both thorns and thistles it shall grow for you'*. Again it is evident that it is the land that is making its own response to Adam in response to his choice. Judgement is not missing from this approach to understanding the Fall. This curse from the ground is a judgement, I am not stepping back from that stark fact. Note, however, that God does not seem to be instigating some all-together new regime of judgement and punishment. He is not setting up the creation as a prison house of divine retribution. Rather, he is speaking to Adam and Eve of the consequences that will now follow from their actions. Divine justice is not foremost in God's mind; rather, his desire is to keep humanity in touch with reality.

God is telling Adam and Eve what is now happening in creation; this with a view to ensuring that they will be able to continue to engage in ongoing correspondence with their finite counterpart – the creation. For if they lose that connection, if the 'language' between them and creation becomes confused, there will be no way for humans to make proper sense of God or creation or, indeed, themselves.

curses and blessings that land

Let's now take a closer look at what that curse in the ground is about. In Scripture the curse is most often used in conjunction with its opposite number – the blessing. Moses said in Deuteronomy 30:19: *'I call heaven and earth to witness against you today, that I have set before you life and death, the blessing and the curse. So choose life in order that you may live, you and your descendants'*. In Scripture, the blessing and the curse are seen to most often come from within the land. In the Genesis 3 account, it was very obvious that the curse arose from the ground. What then might a land that was blessed look like? Of Joseph, God said, *'Blessed of the Lord be his land, with the choice things of heaven, with the dew, and from the deep lying beneath'* (Deut. 33:13). This and other similar verses speak of the bounty and richness that come from a land blessed by God. To me, this speaks of the *'fullness'* that Paul refers to in Ephesians 1:23. The same is in view in the Gen. 1:28 phrase: *'fill the earth'*. This earth, the ground of our existence, *'is the Lord's and the fullness thereof'* (Ps. 24:1 AV), containing everything from *'the choice things of heaven'* to the riches of *'the deep lying beneath'*.

It is evident from these and other Scriptures that post-Fall we do not just have the curse. Instead, we now have the blessing and the curse. It is very important that we grasp this part of creation reality. Spurred on by Plato, too many theologians have turned the creation into the curse itself, as if creation is now commensurate with that curse. Not true! There is a curse that arises in and from the ground, but the curse is not the ground itself. This approach gives room for that ground to hold within it the capacity for both the curse and the blessing.

So what is a curse? Well, if the blessing is a power that releases the good bounty of creation into one's life, it would follow that the curse would be a power that hinders (or stops) one's ability to gather the bounty (ie the good fruits of creation) into that life. This is first-base in understanding this particular force of creation. Second base, in regards to the curse, has to do with creation's capacity to send a payload of consequences into the body of those who go against the grain of the good in life. In this regard, note Jeremiah 23:10: *'for the land is full of adulterers; for the land mourns because of the curse. The pastures of the wilderness have dried up. Their course also is evil, and their might is not right'*.

If we continue to do that which is against God, and thus against life, then the curse within the land can impact on our body and our mind. This rather stark consequence, arising from the curse, is very much in view in Deuteronomy chapter 28. We will look in some detail at the blessings and cursings portrayed in this chapter when we come to consider the role of disease and death in the remedial space design of creation in chapter eleven of this book.

one judgement, lots of consequences

When God made the creation he said it was good, very good. It was this goodness that we were born to gather into our life, work and worship. When we think of the thorns, sweat and death that arose or were multiplied at the time of the Fall, it does seem that God wanted to punish us by cursing the creation. But again, if we focus on the creation of God and his ongoing purpose for our lives, we might begin to see a different picture emerge. Imagine what would have happened to the human race, post-Fall, if the full measure of God's bounty and blessing had remained fully accessible to humans, and particularly, to evil humans. If such were the case, the extent of human evil and misery would have been far greater than it has been throughout human history.

In that light, consider this: at the time of the Fall the full measure of the good that God placed in creation (ie *'the fullness'*) was safeguarded behind the barriers put in place in response to Adam and Eve's sin; these being the thistles and thorns that made work more difficult; the reduced yield from the introduction of the curse in the ground; and, finally, the decay and ultimate death of the human body (which we will soon consider). What say if God designed these 'consequential' forces to ensure that no one human (nor humanity in general) could fully access the measure of the 'creation goods'. I think it's a thought worth thinking. In this regard, note the following graphic.

Post Fall Womb of Creation:
thorns, sweat, death

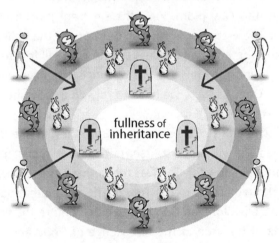

To bring creation reality to bear on a person's state of being so as to restore, preserve and promote his/her health and well-being is a good thing. To intervene so as to stop the spread of a disease or a cancer and thereby save a life is a good thing. To safeguard life by putting in place a vast 'creation immune system' that resists pathogens that would otherwise colonise and destroy the body is a good thing. All of these constitute good therapeutic practice. All of these things I believe God did for and on behalf of humanity. We will consider more of these 'good' effects of the Fall as we proceed. For now, let's make a move to the next consequence of Adam and Eve's decision to sin – that being death.

the meaning of death

God said of Adam and Eve that *'by the sweat of your face you shall eat bread till you return to the ground, because from it you were taken; For you are dust, and to dust you shall return'*. Surely, one might say, this death must be a judgement. After all, did not God say in relation to the Tree of Good and Evil that *'in the day that you eat from it you shall surely die'* (Gen. 2:17)? Let's consider.

First of all, if this phrase had to do with divine punitive justice for sin, then one might have expected a quick execution of the only two people on earth – finito! But no, the only thing killed on that day was an animal whose coat was required to douse their ruddy shame. The word *'death'*, when used in Scripture, refers to the act of separation – the life from the body (Mk. 15:39), the person from the Law (Rom. 7:4), the sin from its consequence (1 Pet. 2:24). Adam and Eve were not immortal. Contrary to the beliefs of the Greek philosophers, and the Pharisees of Jesus' time who fell for them, humans do not possess an immortal soul. We are contingent beings made of clay and breathed into by God. As such, we have to rely on a constant source of God's life-breath to exist.

When Adam and Eve chose against God, they, in effect, chose against life. They still had life within, of course, but their relationship with God had changed. The problem now for God was that as long as they were in Eden they would have continued access to the Tree of Life, a tree that had the ability to keep their bodies alive forever. God had decided before the Fall that if Adam and Eve partook of the Tree of the Knowledge of Good and Evil they would die. Now that such a course had been chosen, God (it seems) had to make a decision as to how this death might come to pass. What followed from there was a conversation within the triune Godhead, with the Father saying, *'"Behold, the man has become like one of Us, knowing good and evil; and now, lest he stretch out his hand, and take also from the tree of life, and eat, and live forever"* —' (Gen. 3:22).

Again, if God had already decided on swift justice ending in death, then why was there a need to have this conversation? There must be something else coming into play here. It is apparent, from the above verse, that God is not focused on bringing death to Adam and Eve. Rather, his concern is that the first couple would continue to live under the Law and its many impacts, physically and spiritually. There is a world of difference between directly killing a person and allowing them to live out their life-span.

So it was that after a long pause at the end of Genesis 3:22, God's voice, it appears, trails off into a silent sadness; as if he could not bring himself to say the words that spoke of premature exile from the Garden. The writer of the Genesis account takes up where God left off, saying: *'therefore the Lord God sent [Adam] out from the garden of Eden, to cultivate the ground from which he was taken'* (Gen. 3:23). It was this decision on the part of God that ensured that Adam and Eve's bodies would in time return to the dust of earth from whence they came. What happened to their soul, however, is quite another matter.

get your deaths right

In the Scriptures we are presented with two distinct facets of the human being; they being the physical body and the spiritual/divine breath. The first account of this human design is found in Genesis 2:7. There we read that *'the Lord God formed man of dust from the ground, and breathed into his nostrils the breath of life; and man became a living being'*. In chapter 12, and vs 7 of Ecclesiastes, we read that when a person dies their *'dust will return to the earth as it was, and [their] spirit will return to God who gave it'*.

I cannot underestimate the importance of this distinction between the body and the soul of human beings. Not only does it help us understand why God did not just kill Adam and Eve on sight when they sinned, but also, it enables us to understand why God, post-Fall, placed a use-by-date on the human body. I will go into some detail in regards to this key distinction between body and soul in chapter seven and onwards.

For now to say, there is no mention in the Genesis 3 account of the Fall of Adam's soul suddenly becoming spiritually dead to God; the same applies to Eve. The death they ultimately died was physical and not spiritual. This understanding of death and the body has, I believe, the potential to transform our reading of Scripture. The New Testament refers to *'death'*, *'dead'*, *'die'* and *'dying'* cumulatively 348 times. For the most part, when Christians read these words they think they are referring to spiritual death with a view to eternal punishment. But what if verses such as Ephesians 2:1, which speak of our being *'dead in [our] trespasses and sins'*, are actually referring to the demise of the physical body. Imagine the shift in our approach to life if we saw these hundreds of references as pointing to the physical body and its use-by date. In particular, for those whose life is given to tending to the ills, decay and death of the human body, imagine how their theology of the body might begin to change. More on this to come.

unusual wrath

It's now time to make sense of what I think is the most unusual thing that happened on that fallen day. It relates to God's words to Eve about the consequences of her own actions. God said to Eve: *'I will greatly multiply your pain in childbirth. In pain you shall bring forth children'* (Gen. 3:16). What is of note here is that God himself has decided to multiply Eve's pain in childbirth; this as distinct from the creation itself responding – as per those thorns and thistles and that curse in the ground. The decision on the part of God to multiply the pain of women in childbirth is, in anyone's estimation, a judgement so strange that it defies reason. When you read, *'I will greatly multiply your pain in childbirth'*, you could read it again and again and still not make much sense of it. If this is divine wrath, then it is very strange wrath indeed!

If, however, you turned to Romans 8 and read verse 22, you could start to get a handle on the redemptive significance of this most telling judgement. Truth is that, not only the woman, but also *'the whole creation groans and suffers the pains of childbirth together until now'*. This begs the question: was Eve's judgement simply a divine punishment or was it one of the most amazing signs of hope and redemption ever given? On my part, I go for the 'hope and redemption' option.

This divine marker of pain in childbirth carries within it the code for what has to happen between humanity and creation. The hope given to Eve by God was that in the fullness of time the pain of a woman's birth pangs (ie Mary) would give birth to the Son of God. This is the Son who would crush the serpent's head, take away the consequences of sin, go through every judgement and consequence of the Fall, and from there, take the journey from death, to life, to earth, through the heavens to the very Throne of God. It is this journey, in Christ, that we must follow; this so that we, as sons and daughters, might take hold of our inheritance in creation (as per Ps. 8), and, thereby, our inheritance in God. It is a lot to say in one or two breaths! That is why, in this book, I will spend considerable space exploring this divine progression;

particularly that last part of the journey I mentioned above – re our following Christ from earth through the heavens.

In this interaction between humanity and pain and death, the devil had no say whatsoever. It was God who sent Adam and Eve into a more hostile and challenging creation; this because it was the best option for humanity. And it was God who set up a situation whereby Adam and Eve would one day die; this, again, because it was the best option for humanity. Also, it was God who decided that pain is not always a bad thing; rather, it is a most powerful sign given to point us in the direction of divine and creation reality. As we shall see in detail in chapter ten, creation's travail has been exquisitely and divinely designed to give birth to creation's *'fullness'* (as per Eph. 1:23).

burning love

After our, I would hope, illuminating visit to Eden, let's reflect on the nature of God. Those from the divine-justice fellowship make much of God's wrath at the time of the Fall. No doubt God was angry when Adam and Eve sinned. But in the account of what happened at that time, God's statements to them seemed considered and direct; rather than boiling over in anger. What then is this anger, this wrath; where does it come from?

God is love, and that infinite love is the ground from which our understanding of wrath must come. When a person you deeply love betrays or rejects you, that now wounded love can very quickly turn into a deep and passionate anger. God was often wounded in love by those he loved. One such instance was recorded in Isaiah 54:8, where God said of Israel that *'in an outburst of anger I hid my face from you for a moment; but with everlasting loving kindness I will have compassion on you.'* Here we discover that in one instance God is eternal in an outburst of anger and in the next moment he is eternal in an outburst of compassion. This indicates to me that we must not freeze-dry any emotion of such a God as this!

which cosmos is yours?

I believe that our loss or lack of understanding of the physical creation God has made has exacted a heavy toll on far too many Christians. In effect, the saints have been taught, for the most part, to (theologically) bypass the present creation and instead focus on a heaven of the afterlife. Thus the challenge – which version of creation reality will we choose? To me, Plato's damaging influence on the church's understanding of the Fall is more than evident. As such, I believe it is way past time we took a cosmological cure from the Hebrews of old.

The Hebrew vision of creation's design and purpose is not some quaint relic of ancient mythology. Rather, it offers a blueprint that will help us make a whole lot more sense of life in God. This ancient Hebraic cosmology has the potential to bring new light and new wisdom to our understanding and experience of creation, which includes the likes of disease, suffering, decay and death.

In the next two chapters I will look into two more facets of the creation design, as understood by the Hebrews of old. The first has to do with the relationship between the heaven of God and the earth. And the second has to do with the material and spiritual design of the creation. These designs will help us establish a larger creation context within which we can more clearly locate and relate to the things and forces God has made. Let's now seek, in mind and heart, to connect the heaven of God to the dwelling place of humans – that being planet earth.

04

Space Time
Heaven Earth

At this stage in the book, some readers might be thinking: 'we have reached the fourth chapter and the author still hasn't told us about how we might apply the Scriptures to our understanding of healthcare and healing'. My first response to these 'thinkers' is to remind them of my words at the end of the first chapter; just in case they read that section a little bit too quickly. My second response is to take opportunity, as Peter the apostle did, *'to stir you up by way of reminder'* (2 Pet. 1:13). In the author's preface, I referred to my hope for this book; which I will now express again, but via different wording.

My hope is that a better understanding of God's creation will enable those who work in healthcare and allied disciplines to discover more about themselves, their relationships and their responses to those who come to them for help and healing. To accomplish this, I believe that Christians in healthcare need to understand more about the nature, design and purpose of God's creation. To succeed in this endeavour we will need assistance from the ancient Hebraic vision of life in God's good creation. So, with these reminders in place, let's now knock on heaven's door and see what the earth does in response to our heavenly plea.

it looks like a plan, but it's really about relationships

As a primer to the theological journey we are about to undertake, I will commence this chapter with the apostle Paul's description of what he calls *'the eternal purpose'*. In Ephesians 3:9-11 the apostle speaks of his mission to bring about an understanding of God's strategy for the church in creation.

His apostolic passion, he says, is *'to bring to light what is the administration [or stewardship] of the mystery which for ages has been hidden in God, who created all things'*. This 'administration' has been put in place, he says, to enact an eternal and strategic plan for humanity. It was established, he says, *'in order that the manifold wisdom of God might now be made known through the church to the rulers and the authorities in the heavenly places'*. This entire plan, Paul says, *'was in accordance with the eternal purpose which [God] carried out in Christ Jesus our Lord'*.

To say the least, there's a lot to take in here! For now, I simply note two things. The first is that the context of these verses has all to do with *'God, who created all things'* – ie the divine plan has to do with God and his creation. The second is that the focus of God's plan for Christ's body, the church, is on *'the rulers and the authorities in the heavenly places'*. It follows from this that if we do not know what creation is and who these rulers are or where these heavenly places are located, then we are going to find it very difficult to work out this divine plan; which is to say, we really need to get our cosmology right!

My intent in this chapter is to bring back (in our minds and our sight) the heaven of God from its Platonic exile, and place it where it is always been – over and around God's good earth. Yes it's true, I literally believe that right now the heaven of God exists in space and time over and around the earth. Some might shut the book on me at this point. Such is their want and their right. For readers who might find this cosmology infantile or embarrassing they can, of course, elect to deem this belief to be simply a metaphor. In this way they might at least be able to continue this exploration.

In a modern-day scientific era, why would I be at pains to re-introduce the idea that God's heaven is around and above all of the earth? Well, to say the least, the 'return' of God's heaven over and around the earth would constitute one very big vote of confidence in the creation. So that's a start. Yes, I am aware that Plato's philosophical and theological offspring would not be happy with such a move as this; they being trained to keep God's pure/eternal heaven a long way away from tainted earth and its fleshly desires. But did not God himself become flesh, so that his plan for humankind might triumph? As such, we need to be aware of what we think, not only about the nature of the human body, but also the entire creation that God has made.

heavenly co-ordinates

Around one hundred verses in Scripture refer directly to the vital relationship between the earth and the heaven of God. The truth is that heaven and earth were made for each other! God's heaven enables us to make sense of his earth (as per Matt. 6:10). As such, if we are confused about the whereabouts of God's heaven, we will also be confused about life and work on planet earth. Again I call to mind Paul's words from 1 Cor. 15:46: *'the spiritual is not first, but the natural; then the spiritual'*. For us humans, it is earth first and then heaven; and if we split or sever them, we are bound to lose our way.

Isaiah knew about this divine blueprint from the very mouth of God, who said: *'Heaven is my throne, and the earth is my footstool'* (Isa. 66:1). Not only is it evident from these words that God's Throne is connected to the earth, but also the very person of God is seen to exist, or be present, from earth all the way through to God's heaven. There is no way we can apply Plato's cosmology to this verse without ending up with a very strange picture of a God whose head is in the afterlife, whilst his severed feet somehow remain on this earthly life – hence my preference for the Hebrew version of divine reality.

SPATIAL AWARENESS

In the *New International Dictionary of New Testament Theology* Vol. 2, the theologian, Colin Brown, says that *'Man has always contrasted heaven with his earthly environment. To the physical relationship there has also corresponded a metaphysical one. As well as being a spatial term, heaven became a general expression for everything that has power over man, the domain of gods and spirits.'* P.184.

I have often looked but could never find any mention in the Bible of God's heaven being located outside of space and time. As such, one wonders why the saints are so committed to a doctrine that has no validation from Scripture. By way of further example of this, I note the author Millard J. Erickson, who wrote a well-known book on Christian theology. In that book he refers to a change that took place in the Western mind from a belief in a flat earth to that of a spherical earth. I am aware that many cultures prior to the scientific revolution did believe the earth was round and not flat; but that is not my concern here. Rather, my interest is in how this theologian locates the heaven of God in this transition from a flat to a spherical earth.

Of God's heaven, Erickson says: *'The biblical conception [of God] depends heavily upon spatial imagery. God is thought of as "higher", "above", "high and lifted up"... In biblical times and for centuries thereafter it was assumed that all heavenly bodies are located in an upward direction from the surface of the earth. But the knowledge that the earth is not a flat surface and is actually part of a heliocentric system which is in turn part of a much larger universe has made this assumption untenable. Further, what an American terms "up" is "down" to an Australian, and vice versa. It will not do, then, to try and explain transcendence in terms of a vertical dimension'*. Christian Theology (Baker Book House, Grand Rapids, Michigan, USA, 5th Printing 1998), p. 313. That's it then, no more heaven over earth for you!

cosmo-logic

Having established a fondness for God's heaven over my earth, I feel the need to go after Erickson's cosmological logic. I believe he is confusing God with God's heaven. Truth is, however, that there is an infinite difference between God and God's heaven. To mistake the two leads to a deep flaw in reasoning. So many times I hear Christians saying that heaven is eternal, as if it has, of itself, that quality of existence. It does not. God is transcendent and eternal, whereas heaven is finite and thus is able to exist in and through space and time. Real space and actual time exist in God's heaven; so much so that in that place there is a form of time-keeping. We read that when Christ *'broke the seventh seal, there was silence in heaven for about half an hour'* (Rev. 8:1). There you have it, half an hour in a finite heaven with finite beasts, elders, angels and seven finite scrolls.

The heaven of God is the place of God's Throne; a throne that exists, not so much for the sake of God himself, but for the sake of humanity. That is why God located this throne – his rule – over the earth. Just as Westminster is the seat of British government, so too the Throne of God is the seat of his rule over the earth. We would, I would hope, never mistake the Westminster building with the prime minister in situ; nor should we mistake God's heaven for God himself!

In summary, to confuse the transcendence of God with the heaven of God, and from there employ this confusion to jettison God's heaven off into some eternal realm on the other side of death, just will not do! All Millard had to do to ensure that Australia did not miss out on heaven was to take a look at Colossians 1:17 and grasp the truth that in God the Son, *'all things hold together'*. This information might then have stirred his imagination to consider that the finite heaven of God also exists *around* the entire earth. This would not only have been a cosmologically consistent approach, but more importantly, it would have served to keep God's heaven in place over and around God's amazing earth.

the heaven of heavens

Let's now dig a little deeper, so as to reach further into God's plan for his heavens over and around his earth. In Ephesians 1:20 Paul says that God has *'seated [Christ] at his right hand in the heavenly places'*. This indicates that Christ is not only seated at God's right hand in the heaven of God, but he also exists (is seated) in and through the other heavens as well. Matthew 5:16 (ILGE), refers to *'the Father of you in the heavens'* – as in *'heavens'* plural. In the Old Testament, and to a lesser degree in the New, the word translated as *'heaven'* is plural, rather than singular. In this regard, I note Psalm 115:16, which says that *'the heavens are the heavens of the Lord; but the earth he has given to the sons of men'*. Here, God is seen as ruling in and through all of the heavens over the earth.

When the writers of the Old Testament referred to this ultimate place of God's rule over the earth, they spoke of the *'heaven of heavens'* (Neh. 9:6) or *'highest heavens'* (1 Kings 8:27). Paul the apostle speaks of being *'caught up to the third heaven'* (2 Cor. 12:2). Two verses on he speaks of being *'caught up into Paradise'* (ibid. vs 4), which is to say that the two are one and the same place. In Revelation 2:7, the Holy Spirit says that *'to him who overcomes, I will grant to eat of the tree of life, which is in the Paradise of God'*.

These verses clearly indicate that Paul believed that *'the third heaven'* was the *'throne of God'* (Heb. 12:2), situated in the highest heaven. I am aware that different apocalyptic writings refer to one, three, five or seven heavens, as well as some adding different levels to each heaven. But for me, Paul's mention of being caught up to *'the third heaven'* – indicating the existence of at least three heavens – is a good enough start-point. So then, what are these two other heavens and what is their relationship to the heaven of God?

As we read Scripture, we are made very much aware of three main players in life: humans on earth (living alongside animals, plants and the like); angels, who are not adverse to turning up at times in great numbers, literally forming *'a multitude of the heavenly host'* (Luke 2:13); and God, the ultimate creator of all things, who has a throne surrounded by a myriad of angels, twenty-four elders, four beasts and one crystal sea. Each of these three players (humanity, angels and God) is seen to be present or, more accurately, have their seat of power in their respective spatial/heavenly realms. Humans have their 'seat' in the atmospheric heavens – that is why God called them to 'rule over the birds of the heaven' (Gen. 1:28). The angelic 'seat of power' in Hebrew cosmology is identified spatially with the planets and the stars – as per the following description.

STAR CELEBRATION

The Hebrews were brought up to see the unseen within the seen. As such they were able to see a light and hear the sound coming down from a far distant time 'when the morning stars sang together, and all the sons of God shouted for joy' (Job 38:7). When they came into Canaan, they welcomed the backup they got from 'the stars [who] fought from heaven... against Sisera' (Judges 5:20). Daniel, one of their prophets, saw a little nation that 'grew up to the host of heaven and caused some of the host and some of the stars to fall to the earth'. So too, Christ spoke of a time when 'the stars will be falling from heaven, and the powers that are in the heavens will be shaken'. As such, should we not, as the offspring of Abraham, also declare: 'is not God in the height of heaven? Look also at the distant stars, how high they are!' (Job 22:12). And to that we might add the cosmological anthem: 'Praise him, sun and moon; praise him, all stars of light!' (Psalm 148:3).

---

one, two, three

From the first heaven to the second, there follows the third. God's heaven is seen as existing beyond the heavens of humanity and angels. This sight gave to the Hebrew people a profound 'spatial' sense of God's presence and rule in and over the vast universe. Yahweh was not some tribal deity – he was and is God 'most high'. For the Western mind this may seem strange. But for the Hebrews of old and many indigenous cultures, the fact that the divine inheres in space and time presents no problem to their mind.

This 'heavenly' relatedness is perhaps mostly succinctly expressed in the following words used to describe Lucifer's bad move: 'you said in your heart, "I will <u>ascend to heaven</u> [God's heaven]; I will raise my throne <u>above the stars of God</u> [angelic heaven], and I will sit on the mount of assembly in the recesses of the north. I will ascend <u>above the heights of the clouds</u> [human heaven]; I will make myself like <u>the Most High</u>"' (Isa. 14:13-14).

In Scripture we are often met by angels coming to earth and apostles and prophets heading to heaven; not to mention certain visits by Lucifer to the Throne of God. This is to say that there is lots of trade and traffic going on between these heavens. On the day of Pentecost *'suddenly there came from heaven a noise like a violent, rushing wind, and it filled the whole house where they were sitting'* (Acts 2:2). A few months later Saul was on his way to Damascus when *'suddenly a light from heaven flashed around him and he fell to the ground'* (Acts 9:3-4). These are not myths. This is the way the Hebrews experienced the power and presence of God's person and rule in their life, work and worship.

This God-given sight enabled the Israelites of old to experience the divine within and through space and time. This psychological and spatial experience empowered them to engage the heaven of God in, through and over their everyday life. They knew that God's Throne was far above and beyond their earth. But at the same time this heaven and its inhabitants could respond to them, in song – *'drip down, O heavens, from above, and let the clouds pour down righteousness; let the earth open up and salvation bear fruit, and righteousness spring up with it. I, the Lord, have created it'* (Isa. 45:8).

revisit your heavens to re-locate your earth

At the outset of this chapter I referred to Paul's description of *'the eternal purpose'*, which is all about *'the manifold wisdom of God... [being] made known through the church to the rulers and the authorities in the heavenly places'*. Again to stress what is at stake here: if we are going to engage and fulfill the above-stated *'eternal purpose'*, we will need to follow both the Hebrew script and the Hebrew vision of all creation under God's heaven. Let's now proceed to the second key design God put in place from *'in the beginning'*; that being the seen/unseen or material/spiritual make-up of God's vast creation; made, of course, with we humans in mind.

05

Sight
of the Unseen

This chapter will require some consideration of a philosophical nature. I would hope that it might bring more clarity, rather than adding confusion to the reader. The premise is simple: that being that the seen/material forms in creation are designed to engage with the unseen/spiritual forms in that same creation. This understanding will help us fathom a lot more of the creation forces that work to serve God's *'eternal purpose'* (Eph. 3:11). It will also help us understand a lot more about our relationship to the infinite and eternal person of God. I would go so far as to say that this seen/unseen revelation of Scripture sits at the core of Paul the apostle's theology. So then, let's unpack this divine payload.

Paul the apostle sent two letters to the troubled Corinthian church. In the second letter he said to them that they should *'look not at the things which are seen, but at the things which are not seen; for the things which are seen are temporal, but the things which are not seen are eternal'* (2 Cor. 4:18). On first reading these words I would imagine that many of the Corinthians might have been a bit confused. Paul, it seems, was suggesting that they should not focus on the seen things, but rather on the unseen things. One could imagine what a Corinthian believer might have done in response to this directive. It's speculation, I know, but consider this: one of those Corinthian believers was at home and had been thinking about this part of Paul's letter, re those seen/ unseen apostolic instructions. Suddenly, he heard the footsteps of his wife and realised that soon she would enter the room – which she did.

She said 'hello', and he said 'nice day'. From there, following Paul's advice, he made sure he did not look at her. Instead, he focused on a vacant space between two water containers.
'What are you doing?' she said.
'Nothing', he said, still looking into space.
'You're up to something', she responded.
There was a silent stand-off for twenty or so seconds, which ended when she said: 'enough with your stupid joke'.
She then clasped her hands around his face and said: 'look at me, or else!'
He knew it was time to follow his wife, and forget the apostle, at least for now!

So, what on earth was Paul thinking when he wrote these words? To find out we will need to take a look at the word *'look'* in the above verse. In the Greek, this word is *skopunton*; its tense being present continuous. If we apply this to the above verse we could read Paul's words this way: *'do not keep looking at the things which are seen, but keep looking at the things which are not seen; for the things which are seen are temporal, but the things which are unseen are eternal'*. It is a light touch, but it makes a lot of difference to what is being communicated here – as per the follow-on account of our Corinthian believer.

After Tuesday night prayers he talked to a church elder, re the issue of the seen and unseen things, as relating to his wife. After hearing the story the elder, supressing his desire to laugh, said: 'No, no; that's not was Paul had in mind. What he is saying is that you should keep engaging the physical form of your wife, so that you can continue to engage her relationally and spiritually'. Many thanks, said the Corinthian.

To further emphasise this seen/unseen design I will combine the verse from Romans 1:20 with what Paul said to the Corinthians. The apostle says that *'since the creation of the world [God's] invisible attributes, his eternal power and divine nature, have been clearly seen, being understood through what has been made'* (Rom. 1:20). Because of this we need to ensure that we do not just *'keep looking at the things which are seen, but [rather] keep looking at the things which are unseen; [ie those invisible attributes, that eternal power and divine nature]*. And why is it that this way of seeing and engaging the creation is so important? It is because *'the things which are seen [the physical/material forms] are temporal [ie they pass away over time], but the things which are unseen are eternal [ie they are, by nature, divine]'* (2 Cor. 4:18). This clearly indicates the significance of the seen/unseen design of creation. What we also notice here is that, for the Hebrews, the unseen dimension is one and the same as the spiritual dimension – eg *'[God's] <u>invisible</u> attributes'* and *'the things which are <u>unseen</u> are eternal'*.

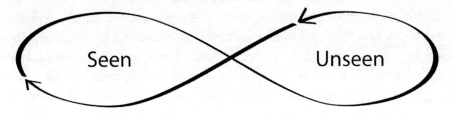

opposites attract

It is very clear from the above verses that the unseen/spiritual dimension exists in some way within the physical forms of creation – and that, of course, for a very strategic and divine reason. Here again we are met with the theological importance of the physical realm in its connection to the spiritual/divine dimension. What comes into focus here is the relationship that is formed between these two facets of creation. Whilst the 'seen' keeps moving towards the 'unseen', so too, the 'unseen' keeps moving towards the 'seen' – as per the above graphic. It is this dynamic movement that generates, upholds and, yes, guides the relationship between the seen/material forms and the unseen/spiritual forms.

In contrast to this, Plato's cosmology severs this relationship; this by making one the opposite or a negation of the other. As much as church leaders tell the saints to not mix the divine (ie God) with the physical creation, they still turn up on Sunday to experience God in and through seen/material things such as preaching, preachers, songs, instruments, candles, communion tables and so on. Apparently it is OK for material forms to mix in with the spiritual or divine dimension, just as long as it happens in a religious setting. For my part, I think we need to establish a much larger common ground, in regards to this issue of God's relationship to material forms. I think that the same rules that apply in the church gathering should be able to apply to all of God's creation, which, of course, is also sacred on the basis of the one who made it. To find this common and sacred ground we will need to be further *'renewed in the spirit of... our mind'* (Eph. 4:23).

mining the seen/unseen paradox

In Proverbs 23:7, we read that *'as [a man] thinks within himself, so he is'*. In this regard, it is of note how peoples' version of reality establishes their patterns of thinking. I have referred to dualism, which creates its own particular 'mind-map'. Another form of thinking is the linear pattern. In this approach the person sees themselves as moving forwards, backwards or stationary on a desired path or progression. For example, God's heaven is seen as being more glorious or divine than the earth below. As such, people desire, in some way, to ultimately progress from earth to heaven – eg Isa. 45:8 and Eph. 4:9-10. As distinct from dualism, I believe that this linear approach is useful to God's purpose.

There is a third pattern of thinking, which I believe is essential to our engagement with God and his creation. I call this a 'paradox pattern'. Paradox was often used by Jesus and Paul. By way of examples: Christ says that *'he who has found his life shall lose it, and he who has lost his life for my sake shall find it'* (Matt. 10:39). Paul speaks of a life in which we are *'unknown yet well-known, as dying yet behold, we live... as sorrowful yet always rejoicing, as poor yet making many rich, as having nothing yet possessing all things'* (2 Cor. 6:9-10). In these instances, paradox is not seen as a contradiction or an absurdity. Rather, it refers to a relationship in which one thing is known or experienced by way of the contrast and contribution of the other. Note in this regard that the *Australian Concise Oxford Dictionary* describes paradox as *'a seemingly absurd or contradictory statement, even if actually well-founded'*. Many indigenous tribes and Eastern cultures employ paradox to help them make sense of life and the divine. Western based civilisations, on the other hand, tend to be more categorical in their approach to understanding reality. As such, paradox does not feature as much in their 'mind maps'.

one who is three

Another good reason why paradox is so important to our understanding of God and his creation is that its origins are to be found in the Trinity. Each person of the Trinity is ever one in that Trinity and in that oneness they express their distinction in relationship to each other. This divine paradox is both the origin and the nature of the 'seen/unseen' creation design; in that 'the seen' is both distinct from 'the unseen', but is also one with 'the unseen' (and vice versa). Again to say, it is this movement between the two (towards and away and towards again) that generates the relationship. Of course, to activate or realise this relationship for the good, humans will need to work together in line with the creation mandate.

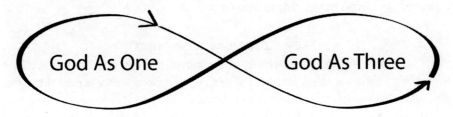

Would it not stand to reason that the same relational design that holds for the Trinity should also apply to *'all things'* God has made? Why would God change the pattern and bring in some other relational reality when this one has worked so long and so well? Hence my belief that the foundational pattern of God's creation design is formed by the 'one with/distinct from' paradox; assisted, of course, by the linear movement.

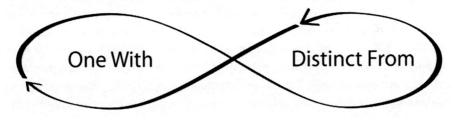

I mentioned the confusion that exists in church culture in regards to the relationship between the spiritual/divine dimension and the material/physical dimension. My conviction is that if we are to end the confusion of Plato's cosmology, we need to take seriously the origins, nature and design of paradox – in God. Truth is that God is able, well able, to be fully one with all created forms and in that relationship remain distinct. He is also the only one that we can be fully one with and in that oneness find our own distinction. So too, God is the only one who can be fully one with us and in that relationship still be distinct from us.

Once we attend to our fear of the physical in our relationship to the divine (this by embracing the one with/distinct from design of reality), we can begin to engage anew with the *'one God and Father of all things who is over all things and through all things and in all things'* (Eph. 4:6 ILGE); this in the knowledge that in, through and over all physical things and forces of creation there exists God's very own attributes, nature and power, every ready to serve us in our growing up in all things into God.

THE PHILOSOPHERS' COMPOUND

Plato did his thing by dividing, in our minds, the unseen from the seen. He then said that the attributes that exist within creation were simply copies of the real attributes that exist in the eternal realm. Aristotle, on the other hand, believed that reality existed within the material realm, with its various attributes being conceptual in form. These conceptual attributes gave rise to classifications, which he said were universal in nature, ie they applied in all circumstances and all times.

St Aquinas was the most prominent theologian of the Scholastic period (circa 1100–1500AD). He and his colleagues eagerly applied Aristotle's universals; particularly so, in regards to their approach to systematic theology, ie putting Bible truths into classifications, eg Christ, church, sin, judgement, salvation and so on. This approach became very popular in the Reformation period. To this day it is still the preferred approach to understanding Scripture in Conservative Evangelical traditions.

Again, what we see here is a world of difference between our two ancient Greeks and the ancient Hebrews. What Paul saw as living and divine attributes in creation (as per Rom. 1:20), these Greeks saw as inanimate *copies* (Plato) and *concepts* (Aristotle) that describe or mirror attributes in the universe. This is the reason why, to this day, most of Christendom thinks that God's invisible attributes, divine nature and eternal power within the physical forms of creation are not living representation of the divine, but rather, they are said to be inanimate sign-posts pointing to a universal idea or a far removed heaven of the afterlife.

If we are to know God and grow in God, we need to 'switch on' in our minds and hearts that which has been 'switched off' by theologians addicted to these Greek cosmologies. It is this shift to an Hebraic cosmology that will enable us to engage the unseen living and divine attributes that reside within the seen forms of God's sacred creation. So, don't let two ancient Greeks steal your inheritance!

creation goods

As I have indicated, this seen/unseen design stands at the heart of Paul's understanding of Scripture. As such, our application of this design will unlock many insights into our life, work and worship in God's creation. By way of example, let's apply this seen/unseen design to the Genesis mandate. God's plan for us humans is that we *'be fruitful and multiply, and fill the earth, and subdue it; and rule over the fish of the sea and over the birds of the sky and over every living thing that moves on the earth'* (Gen.1:28). God ended each of his six days of work with the words, *'it was good'*. And on the seventh day he declared his finished product to be *'very good'*. What we see here is God forming the physical (seen) creation and, as he does, he invests the quality or nature of the (unseen) good into that creation. Let's see how this relationship between the seen/unseen impacted on the first humans.

Before Eve emerged, Adam was told to work the *'garden of Eden [so as] to cultivate it and keep it'* (Gen. 2:15). This work, of course, enabled him to relate to both living and inanimate nature. When Eve came along the number and nature of his relationships were dramatically increased, ie one became two. What we note in this (almost) everyday activity is the two parts that constitute human work. The first is the physical work itself, ie the 'seen/material' forms, and the second is the unseen/relational dimension that arises from that work.

Yes, this is a simple observation, but don't be fooled by its everyday familiarity; the reason being that it holds a key to understanding all relationships between humans, creation and God. What we see here is the means by which human work and the relationships it establishes are able to draw out those Genesis qualities of the 'good', eg God's unseen attributes, nature and power (as per Rom. 1:20), into the life of the worker.

A good example of this process is found in Colossians 1:9-10. The verse begins with *'the knowledge of [God's] will'*. From there we are encouraged to apply God-given *'spiritual wisdom and understanding'* to our chosen endeavour. This assists us to *'walk in a manner worthy of the Lord, [so as] to please him in all things'*. It is this way of life and wisdom that enables us to *'bear... fruit in every good work'*; and it is this fruit (seen and unseen) that leads us *'increasing [into] the knowledge of God' [himself]'*. All this to say that all of our good work in creation is ultimately designed to bring us closer to God. Long live the sacredness of good work!

apostle called up to third heaven

By way of further application of the seen/unseen design, I note again the Hebrew vision of the three heavens – humanity, angelic and God's Throne. Why is it that God made these heavens as they are? Let's explore it.

In the first heaven over the earth we saw how the seen forms of creation held within them the unseen forms, ie attributes – as per Rom. 1:20. When it comes to the angels of the second heaven they are, for the most part, unseen. Yes, they can materialise at times, so as to do their work, and occasionally they take the form of humans. They are, however, more at home to show their unseen face via winds and flames of fire – as per Heb. 1:7. As I said in the previous chapter of this book, the angelic hosts are often identified or associated with planets and stars. So then, there's a lot less *seen/material* forms in the second heaven.

When it comes to the third heaven, the place of God's Throne, we are presented with a realm that has no physical correlate, as in there are no physical/material forms that act as a counterpart to the third heaven. Of course, God can make the unseen visible in a vision to people (eg John's Revelation), but this manifestation is transitory; its form being image-like, as distinct from a physical form. Again the question: why this movement from seen/unseen to less seen/ unseen to entirely unseen?

> 'By faith he [Moses] left Egypt, not fearing the wrath of the king; for he endured, as seeing him who is unseen'
> Hebrews 11:27

Christ knew why. It was he who told us that *'God is spirit [ie unseen], and [as such] those who worship him must worship in spirit and truth'* (John 4:24). This is to say that God planned the heavens as they are so that we might learn to progressively engage the person of God, who is *'eternal, immortal, invisible'* (1 Tim. 1:17). To think, if we had not known the importance of the seen/unseen design, we may well have missed the significance of this key part of ancient Hebraic cosmology.

get your theological bags ready for travel

In chapter three of this book I briefly referred to the journey we need to take from earth through the heavens to the Throne of God; it being akin to the journey Christ took in his life, death and resurrection, from the ground of earth, through to the highest heaven of God. Such being the case, those three heavens must each have a particular role in getting us there. As such, let's keep an eye on these three heavens as we proceed from here; so as to ensure we do not miss any one of their contributions to our cosmic trek from earth to heaven. I will refer to this amazing journey a number of times throughout this book.

I would imagine that some readers would have been faced with a few new concepts in this chapter. To say again, at this stage it is more important to get the picture than it is to get all the points, ie concepts. With the 'heavens over earth' and 'seen/unseen' designs now in place, we are well situated to engage more of the creation territory that God has set before us.

In the next chapter we will be looking to restore, in our hearts and minds, the links between the pre-Fall Eden and post-Fall creation. This will bring us closer to the origins and nature of those creation forces that bring about human pain, disease, decay and death – all of which, of course, are ever present in everyday healthcare and healing practice. So, back to Eden we go.

06

Restoring the Life-links to Eden

Most Christians have been taught to think that the Garden of Eden was a perfect place of no pain, no struggle, not much work and very little stormy weather. As such, it is no wonder that their fairy-tale-like patch of bliss called Eden has very little or no connection to the now (apparently) cursed and spoiled post-Fall creation.

So as to nail my own flag to the mask early in the piece, my belief is that the creation forces of pain, decay, death and, yes, disease existed in some form in pre-Fall Eden. When I say this to Christians most all of them are aghast at the idea. They cannot believe that pain and death existed in the pre-Fall Garden of Eden. To validate this, many cite Revelation 21:4, which says that God *'shall wipe away every tear from their eyes; and [that] there shall no longer be any death; there shall no longer be any mourning, or crying, or pain'*. This passage, which speaks of the age to come, is somehow backdated into the Garden and then viewed as the way things must have been back there in Eden. For all kinds of reasons the beginning of the story is not our goal. We are not seeking a paradise we have lost. We are seeking a much greater place and purpose, based on what Christ has won for us.

I believe we need to update our understanding of Eden, particularly in regards to its relationship to the present creation. To do this I will demonstrate the existence of a number of creation forces that we identify with the Fall, but in fact existed prior to the Fall. Our first force of nature is the Law of God. Of course, those who read the Scriptures are very aware of the significance of the Law. What often seemed strange to me, however, was that something as important as the Law did not get a mention at the time of the Fall. I asked myself – why not?

It was when I dared to take this law down from the high and lofty courts of divine justice and place it *'first... [in] the natural'* (1 Cor. 15:46) that I realised the answer to my question. The Law did not warrant a mention in Eden because from in the beginning, as it is now, the Law is implicit in all things. The Law did not appear from the sky soon after Adam's sin. Rather, it is a dynamic power woven into the very fabric of God's creation.

This is why Adam and Eve felt shame before God came to confirm their guilt. What they felt the instant they chose against God was the force of law arising in their body in response to their sinful action. As Paul says, from the beginning *'the law [was] written in [people's] hearts, their conscience bearing witness, and their thoughts alternately accusing or else defending them'* (Rom. 2:15).

THE LAW: PAST, PRESENT AND FULFILLMENT

Yes, we do read in Scriptures of a time when *'the Law came in'* (Rom. 5:20). But this has to do with the coming of the Mosaic Law, so as to establish the moral, religious and societal laws within the nation of Israel. It was the moral law that continued into the New Covenant, ie Christ's coming. Again to say, this moral law existed long before Israel became a nation – indeed, it existed from the very beginning of God's creation. As Paul says in Rom. 2:14, *'Gentiles who do not have the Law do <u>instinctively</u> the things of the Law'*. This is why *'all who have sinned without the Law will also perish without the Law, and all who have sinned under the Law will be judged by the Law'* (ibid 2:12).

The Law has a *'seen'* form, which is the physical force of cause and effect. And it has an *'unseen'* form, which is the spiritual and relational dynamic of action and consequence. As I said, this law did not suddenly come into existence at the time of the Fall. Rather, it simply responded to the 'down side' of that law, activated by the sin of Adam and Eve. God's law was present in pre-Fall Eden, ever-ready and willing to respond to human actions, be they good or bad.

It was the elemental force of law, this primal dynamic instilled in creation by God, which gave rise to the curse and the blessing in the ground. It was the same force of law within the human conscience that triggered the ground to grow thorns and thistles – *'for you'* Adam. It is the Law that links human pain arising from thorns and thistles to suffering in the *'inner man'*. It also connects the unyielding ground to the sweat and frustration of our labour. Further to this, the Law works to join the good we desire (as per 2 Thess. 1:11) with the good in all things. As such, it is any wonder that this law has to keep going and going *'till all [things] be fulfilled'* (Matt. 5:18 AV). It is this law, under God, which frames the forces that make for the remedial space design of creation.

Oh... the multiplied pain

So then, let's explore the (possible) links between the pre-Fall action and post-Fall forces of pain, decay, death and disease. Was there pain in pre-Fall Eden? Well, that's easy to find out. God said to Eve that he *'will greatly multiply your pain in childbirth'* (Gen. 3:16). It follows logically from this that if there was no pain in childbirth prior to the Fall, there would be no capacity for that pain being multiplied by God. As such, pain must have existed prior to the Fall. Consider this: Adam, pre-Fall, walking along the garden path, hits his foot on a rock. Does he cry out to Eve or does he not – as in, is he in pain? To me it would make sense that Adam would have experienced some form of pain. Had it been a pleasure sensation then most of the creatures of instinct, as well as the first couple, would definitely have got the wrong message about cuts and bruises.

We cannot and should not draw a line between pain that we think is evil and pain that tells us to remove our hand from a fire. Of course, someone might do something bad to us that cause us pain. But it was the action, not the pain, which is the evil in this instance. If we are to work with pain, then we must not split it down the middle; approaching it as an evil on one hand, whilst on the other hand listening to what it is signalling to us in regards to what is going on in the body. Such an approach leads to confusion. It can cause us to create a division between the person and their suffering, thinking that their pain is something 'other' to who they are and what they are going through.

Dr Chris Hayes
Pain Management Specialist, Newcastle, Australia

---

things that wither and die

And what then of death in pre-Fall Eden? As I said in chapter three, the word *'death'*, when used in Scripture, conveys the concept of separation, eg the spirit (or breath) from the body. One cannot, of course, be entirely certain how death was understood or experienced before the Fall. However, the concept, at least, was known to Adam and Eve before the Fall. God said to them that *'from the tree of the knowledge of good and evil you shall not eat, for in the day that you eat from it you shall surely die'* (Gen. 2:17). They could have understood death as simply the opposite of the life they had. However, to my mind, it would have been difficult for Adam and Eve to understand a concept like this unless they saw some representation of it in the creation around them.

One such representation would have been all of those seed-bearing plants that were spoken of in Genesis 1. For a plant to bring forth the next generation of seed, the flower that produces that seed has to wither and 'die'. It has to 'separate' from the plant so that one phase can give way to the next, thus ensuring the ongoing multiplication and survival of the species (as per John 12:24). In this regard, it is of note that animals and organisms in Eden did not have access to the Tree of Life – it being particularly associated with humans in relation to their continuity of life in God. When Adam and Eve no longer had access to that Tree, they began their journey into physical decay and death.

This indicates that animals and organisms, pre-Fall, must have always had a limited life-span – they not having access to that Tree of Life. If such was the case, then, pre-Fall, there would have been many representations of death in both plants and animals. This understanding and experience of decay and death would have formed a key part of Adam and Eve's apprenticeship; equipping them for that time when they would head out beyond the gate and into the wild untamed creation. What then of disease, pre-Fall?

creation's little adversarial allies

Was Adam created with an immune system? If not, then he must have got it after the Fall. There's no record of that, but such could be true – or not. There are no instances of coughs, colds or other infections in the pre-Fall record. Post-Fall, however, the existence of diseases is well and truly in view in Scripture. I have indicated my preference, which is to see the pre-Fall reality as setting in place a continuity of context for the post-Fall period. This then, for me, would place some infections within the Garden gate, arising, perhaps, from those stubbed toes I referred to. In regard to this I note the entry into the Garden of one very dangerous pathogen and predator – that being the serpent. It appears that the Garden was not an entirely safe place after all!

At the beginning of creation there were many forces at play to bring humanity to maturation in God. To rule over the works of God's hands, humans would have to overcome and subdue these forces, which include the fish of the sea, the animals of the land and the birds of the heaven; not to mention those trillions upon trillions of little organisms that lurk in the dirt, ever eager to do business with the human body. If there were no creational forces set against humanity, be they physical or psychological, then the body and soul of Adam and Eve's offspring would have atrophied to jelly. The creation is made of allies and adversaries, forces for and forces against humanity. Both have their place in bringing our immune system (along with us) to a maturity that will enable us to keep engaging the seen and unseen dimensions of these powerful creation forces. Oh yes, and do remember that these things and forces form a key part of your inheritance in God – as per Gen. 1:28.

dualism and the death of human nature

Let's now enquire into the links between Adam and Eve's pre-Fall nature and post-Fall nature. In chapter one I mentioned two doctrines that declare that every human is born spiritually dead to God and sinful by nature. Here follows a popular and long-held explanation of this sad sorry state of all post-Fall humans; this from the *Reformed Westminster Confession of Faith, 1646, Chapter IX, Of Free Will.*

Man, by his fall into a state of sin, hath wholly lost all ability of will to any spiritual good accompanying salvation; so as a natural man, being altogether averse from that good, and dead in sin, is not able, by his own strength, to convert himself, or to prepare himself thereunto.

Not much room to move from there – except, I suppose, into predestination! In chapter three of this book, I referred to the Genesis account of the Fall and noted that at no time in that account did God say anything about us humans being born spiritually dead; nor was there any indication by God at that time that suggested that humans are born sinful by nature. These long-held Reformed ideas are simply not to be found in the foundational Genesis account; nor are they to be found in the rest of the Bible text.

If only these Protestants had distinguished between the seen/ physical forms and the unseen/spiritual forms, they would not have become so confused. But they did not distinguish, and so mistook physical death as spiritual death. From there they added insult to injury by declaring that human nature, made in God's own image and likeness (Gen. 1:27), was at one moment in time changed, so as to become sinful by nature. Who are they that dare declare such a thing as this when there is no validation for it from the Bible text?

WHERE SINGS MY SOUL?

I remember the early years of my being a Christian, having come to Christ in a Pentecostal tradition. During that time my church leaders informed me that my non-Christian soul had been made spiritually dead to God and that on my conversion to Christ I was given a new spirit within my body. I was never quite sure if this spirit was the Holy Spirit or just a brand new human spirit. Yes, I was pleased the get a new spirit, but at times I would wonder what happened to my old soul; as in where was it now?

When I asked my church leaders about this, their main response was to say that my old soul was now sinful by nature and tied to what they called 'the flesh'. But again, they could not tell me where my old soul had gone. Of course I knew that my soul was still me, but in some strange theological way it was not really me – it being by nature sinful. Knowing this, I knew that if I wanted to converse with my old soul it would most probably tell me lies, which would lead me to those sins of the flesh.

Often late at night or when walking along a beach I would hum the tunes to old songs I used to sing during my more pagan/atheistic period. The old soul would often sing along. When this happened, it was like I was visiting a friend who was in prison for crimes, which he did not actually commit – or did he? If my old soul sin nature was an instrument, it would have been a harmonica.

I was walking along a beach in Malaysia in 1980, having done an outreach concert with a music band, and I said to God that I was going crazy. Was I my old soul? Who is my spirit? What was the role played by my flesh? Who is in charge of my mind? And why was it that demons can possess my soul, but not my spirit? I told God that I couldn't put up with this anymore, that it was not working for me. I almost lost my faith, but I kept praying in hope that this confusion would somehow stop. It was during that time that I felt to engage the Hebrew's idea of Scripture and put paid to Plato's confounded dualism.

---

simple fits of faith

The origins of the above cosmological confusion are not just in Pentecostalism. Rather, they arise from beliefs that arose in the early centuries of the Christian church. The Reformed Protestant stream, responsible for the wording of the Westminster Confession, has simply sharpened the edges of what I believe to be Plato's version of the Fall.

There is a much simpler way to understand what happens when a person comes into Christ. And it goes like this: they come out from under *'the Law of sin and of [physical] death'* (Rom. 8:2) and at the same time they come out from under the headship of *'the first man, Adam'* (1 Cor. 15:45). From there, they enter into the headship of Christ, *'the last Adam'* (ibid). In all of this action, the soul, breathed into us by God, remains intact in the human body, with no need of any replacement spirit – as in, no change in human nature. I think that is a simply divine fit; one that enables us, post-Fall, to continue to live in line with a nature that is *of the divine*.

LOW AND BEHOLD, SECOND DEATH FOLLOWS FIRST DEATH

In Ecclesiastes we read that when a person dies their body, as dust, returns *'to the earth as it was, and the spirit will return to God who gave it'* (Ecc. 12:7). From there, in time, they along with all humanity will *'appear before the judgement seat of Christ, so that each one may be recompensed for his deeds in the body, according to what he has done, whether good or bad'* (2 Cor. 5:10). In Rev 2:11 we read that those who are worthy of eternal life *'will not be hurt by the second death'*.

The phrase, *'second death'*, clearly indicates that the death of the body is the first death. Apart from that there are no other deaths on offer. Jesus mentioned this *'second death'*, saying in Matt. 10:28: *'Do not fear those who kill the body but are unable to kill the soul; but rather fear him who is able to destroy both soul and body in hell'*.

---

good medicine, without side effects

We surely need to heal our minds, so as to restore the life-lines that God has set in place for us. I believe that if we do not, we will continue, as Christians, to drift without a firm anchor in the natural realm, with the consequences being that the church as congregation will continue its trend to self-imposed cultural oblivion. Our beginnings are in Eden, and we need to know our beginnings; lest we lose our way on that great journey from earth through creation to God's heaven.

There is a continuity of movement and purpose from the Garden of Eden, through the post-Fall era, all the way to *'the tree of life which is [now apparently resident] in the Paradise of God'* (Rev. 2:7), ie God's heaven. This is why access to that Tree of Life was taken away, lest we had stayed in that old Garden state and not gone out into our inheritance in God's good and wild creation; *'an inheritance which is imperishable and undefiled and will not fade away, [it being ultimately] reserved in heaven for you'* (1 Pet. 1:4).

There is more to know and lots more to do before we arrive at that divine destination; but at least, I would hope, we are moving closer to a better comprehension of the creation, our inheritance. In the next four chapters I will continue our enquiry into the strategic relationship between humans and their counterpart, the creation. This will lead us into chapter eleven, where we will explore in detail the remedial space design of God's amazing creation. I will sign off on this chapter with the following thought.

A WORKING DEFINITION OF HEALTH

Health is about being in right and true relationship with others, with creation and with God. These relationships are designed by God to grow, bringing us into a maturity that will ultimately enable us, in the age to come, to enter into our rule over a renewed created order. As such, in this age, health is not necessarily the absence or presence of disease or infirmity. Indeed, at times disease or infirmity can be used by God as a part of the healing process to bring the individual into right and true relationships with others, with creation and, thereby, with God himself.

––––––––––––––––––––

07

The Divine Design of Human Bodies

It is obvious, I know, but it needs be said: it is human beings who present to healthcare workers asking for help, for a cure, for relief and more. All that happens to these people happens because of events and forces that occur in the creation God has made – again obvious. What is also self-evident is that most all of the focus of the medical system is on the human body. Such being the case, it behoves those who believe in God the creator to have some kind of theological understanding, not just of the body, but also of the entire person.

In chapter two of this book I referred to Dr Meredith Long and her ongoing challenge in regards to engaging what she called 'God's curse' on creation. For her, it seemed that all one could do was to alleviate the effects of this divine curse; as in, make the best of this cursed situation in the hope of one day it will all be over. If I were to express this state of affairs from a graphical viewpoint, I would see an underlying thick, black, almost impenetrable layer of wrath, cursings and punishments that we have to deal with throughout life; and to make this bearable, we need to put in place a pasty white layer over the black, so as to help us compensate for the ongoing burden of that dark/dense part of life.

The dominant focus on punitive justice in regards to the Fall has made it very difficult for us to reach into that sin-filled layer of wrath. As such, it is extremely hard for Christians to make sense of the creation forces that arose or were multiplied at the time of the Fall. In this chapter and the following, I want to reach into this 'miry clay', with a view to releasing four key words of Scripture from its grip – they being the *'flesh'*, *'lust/desires'*, *'instincts'* and *'corruption'*.

First up, to say, these well-known and well-worn words of Scripture have most all to do with the human body, which we will now explore (theologically) in some depth. We begin by taking a look at what makes a human.

breath n dust

In Genesis we are told that the human body was fashioned by God from the 'stuff-n-dust' of creation. From there, a finite measure of God's breath breathed life into that vessel of clay, which gave rise to the existence of the human soul. Why did God make us like this? He could have made the human body out of nothing, *ex nihilo*, but instead he chose to fashion it from the elements he had already made. Why would the infinite God of all creation do such a thing?

I would say that God did this so that the human body could serve as an interface, ie a connection, between the rest of creation and the human soul/spirit. To say it another way, in line with that 'one with/distinct from' paradox motif, our body is one with the creation but distinct within that creation; also our body is one with our *'inner man'* but distinct from that inner man – as per the following graphic.

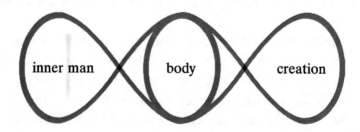

And why would God want this connection to happen? Well, my guess is that it must have something to do with his eternal purpose for humans in creation. In 2 Cor. 4:16, Paul describes one of the consequences of the first sin; that being that *'though our outer man is decaying... our inner man is being renewed day by day'*. Here the *'outer man'* is the physical body (the seen) and the *'inner man'* is the consciousness or life-breath within and through that body (the unseen).

Paul refers to this *'inner man'* as the *'the soul'* (Rom. 2:9) or *'the spirit'* (Rom. 8:10) or *'mind'* (Rom. 7:25) of the person. I am not an advocate of dividing the inner person into spirit and soul compartments. God is spirit (John 4:24), but has a soul (Leviticus 26:11). There is, however, no division in the nature of God. By way of example, we are called to *'love the Lord [our] God with all [our] heart, and with all [our] soul, and with all [our] mind'* (Matt. 22:37). This speaks of one nature, with various attributes that, though distinct, are ever one.

As I have said, for the Hebrew, the word, *'unseen'* is a synonym for the word *'spiritual'* – this in line with 2 Cor. 4:18: *'the things which are <u>not seen</u> are <u>eternal</u>'*. God is eternal and *'God is spirit'* (Jn. 4:24). As such, the inner person, breathed into by God, is, by nature *spiritual*. It follows from this that all relationships between people (and, of course, God) are *of a spiritual* nature – be they good, bad or indifferent in their intent and/or actions.

who sinned, this man or his body?

With this seen/unseen make-up of the person in view, let's now begin to enquire into the nature and location of human sin. In Rom. 7:22-23 Paul the apostle says: *'I joyfully concur with <u>the Law of God in the inner man</u>, but I see a different law in the <u>members of my body</u>, waging war against the Law of my mind, and making me a prisoner of <u>the Law of sin which is in my members</u>'*. In regards to his sin, Paul goes so far as to say that *'now, no longer am I the one doing it, but sin which dwells in me'* (Rom. 7:17).

My first response to this is to not let my young children read this last verse; the reason being that next time they are caught red-handed they might quote it to their mother and claim apostolic immunity! Apart from that concern, it seems to me from Paul's words that he believes that sin resides in the human body; as distinct from sin residing in the *'inner man'*.

Many commentators on this Romans 7 passage have laboured long to make sense of Paul's words written above. In particular, the idea that human have two parts to their nature (as per Rom. 7:22-23 above) is seen by many as a form dualism. In response to that I mention again the critical difference between distinctions that create relationship and divisions that sever them.

Paul, in Rom. 7, was mining the interface between soul and body; carefully distinguishing between the two; and that, it seems, for a very good reason. So the question is asked: why does Paul place sin in the body, and not (it seems) in the entire human person? To find out why, we need to cover some more scriptural ground. In 2 Cor. 5:10, the apostle says that *'we must all appear before the judgement seat of Christ, so that each one may be recompensed for his <u>deeds in the body</u>, according to what he has done, whether <u>good or bad</u>'*. It appears from this verse that the human body not only contains sin, but it also holds within it the good things we do.

My first response to this verse is to say that it stands in contradiction to the idea (or doctrine) that we humans are born *'altogether averse from [the] good and dead in sin* – as per the *Westminster Confession*. One of these doctrinal positions is true, and the other is not. I am further assisted in this choice by the above verse, which informs me that the human body has been designed to convey information that will one day be presented before the very Throne of God. If the human body is sinful by nature, how could God trust it to be an arbiter of human destiny at the end of this age?

It appears to me that God does have some trust in *'the flesh'*. As I indicated in chapter four, the Son of God *'became flesh'* (Jn. 1:14), the same flesh that we are clothed with in this day. So beware what you say about the human body. If God gets all this useful information about life via a read-out from the flesh, then we should follow his lead and take hold of some of that *'manifold wisdom'* (Eph. 3:10) he has placed within it – hence our inquiry into the nature and purpose of the human body.

wild horses

Let's now add to the mix another thing that God was pleased to place in the human body. To find out what this is we turn again to Paul's experience. To the Corinthians he said: *'I buffet my body and lead it as a slave'* (Cor. 9:27 ILGE). One wonders who or what might be buffeting this apostle? Now that we know the body contains both good and bad things within, we cannot say it is just sin or the sin nature getting the better of Paul. Also, would it not be strange if Paul was to be seen walking around Corinth so as to *'lead [his sin] as a slave'*! So, what's it to be?

The word *'buffet'* (in the above verse) suggests to me the act of subduing. Also, the word *'slave'* indicates that someone or something is being ruled over. This reminds me of the Genesis mandate – as per Gen. 1:28 and Psalm 8. Knowing that the human body is *of the creation*, and distinct from the inner person, we can now grasp the truth that Paul is actually wrestling with the creation forces of his own body – these forces being the instincts of his flesh.

This understanding will lead us into many new (and old) insights into the human person. Let's start with one. That which is formed from the physical creation, ie the human body, animals, plants and minerals, is not capable, of itself, to engage in moral or ethical reasoning or choice. It follows from this that the human body, along with the creatures of instinct and other physical/material forms, cannot, of themselves, engage in sin. To put it succinctly, the human body, of itself, cannot sin, it being by nature morally neutral. This, of course, leads us to conclude that it is the inner person that makes the choices for the good, the bad and the in-between, ie it is the inner person that sins, and not the body.

mind your distinctions

Yes, I know that Paul seems of the opinion that sin takes place in the body, rather than in the soul. As such, my statements in the prior paragraph might well be contradicting him. But consider the following story: two thieves devise a plan in a room; that plan being to rob a bank. At this stage in the game they have not yet done the deed. Two days later, however, they go to the bank and steal the money and off they run. A few days later they are caught and thrown into jail – along with the all the money, and the bank and all of its employees. This, to my mind, seems to be a rather strange approach to law and order – is it not?

So too, I think it is strange how theologians can believe that just because sinful actions take place in the body, that it somehow means that the body is, of itself, sinful. When robbers steal money, the money is not viewed as an accessory to the crime. In the same way, sinful actions that take place in and from the body do not make that body sinful in itself. What Paul was saying in Romans 7, in regards to sin in the body, was that the *act* of sin takes place in the body. Such is the case because there is no way or means by which the soul can itself accomplish good or bad deeds. For obvious reasons, there are no hands or eyes in the mind itself!

SIN LOCATIONS

In regards to Romans 7, re the location of sin, I would also say that Paul was at pains to teach the saints to distinguish between the body and the soul; particularly in regards to the movement of their soul out from Adam and into Christ. Paul wanted them to know that their Adamic body was subject to 'the law of sin and of death' (Rom. 8:2), but that also there was another 'law of God [that operates] in the inner man [ie the soul]' (Rom. 7:22) in Christ. If this distinction between body and soul had collapsed into one 'muddle', then Christians would have become very confused about where they stood in life and in God.

Such is the radicalness of this change of standing in creation, that Paul is able to say, in regards to his sin, that *'I [in Christ] am no longer... the one doing it, but sin [in Adam's body] which indwells me'* (Rom. 7:17). Yes, it comes across as being extreme, but Paul needed to let believers know that, among all of the challenges of the Adamic body, their inner person existed in God the Son made human. This apostolic approach in Rom. 7, re sin, is, of course, tempered by many other verses that speak of our responsibility for sin in the body.

———————————————

here sings my soul

I stop here for the moment so as to rejoice in the theological spoils of insight we have gathered. In line with the seen/unseen design, we can now take hold of the truth that, instead of us humans being sinful by nature, we are in fact made up of a body that is instinctual by nature (it being *of creation*). Further to this, we can also declare that our soul, from birth, has been and still is divine by nature (as per Gen. 1:26). This, to me, is a theological game changer. It is enough, I would hope, to cause a *reformation* of sorts in that old Westminster Confession! Let's now begin to trade on this wise-old information.

In 2 Pet. 2:10, the apostle refers to people *'who indulge the flesh in its corrupt desires'*. Two verses down, Peter goes on to say that such people are *'like unreasoning animals, born as creatures of instinct to be captured and killed'* (ibid 2:12). The ILGE version of this last verse reads as follows: *'these men, without reason, like animals, having been born natural for capture and corruption'*.

When Christians read such words or phrases, as per the above two verses, the tendency is to think that every third word is referring to sin; as in, the flesh is sin, desires/lusts are sin, instincts are sin and corruption is sin. From our seen/unseen enquiry, however, we now know that none of these creation forces (as underlined above) are sinful in themselves. The only references in these verses to the act of sinning is the word, *'indulge'*, and the phrase, *'like unreasoning animals'*.

a piece of paper cannot eat itself

Think for a moment about the idea that human desire is an expression of the sin nature. If such were true, then there would be no distinction between indulging the flesh (as per 2 Pet. 2:10) and human desire itself, ie they would be one and the same thing – that being *of sin*. But how can that work in reality?

There is no way in God's good universe that an instinctual desire can exist whilst perpetually consuming itself (ie indulging in itself). If such was the case, then black holes would have swallowed the universe long before it had ever begun! As in, it's an impossibility.

For sin or righteousness to exist, there needs to be other forces and forms that act in response to them. These forces, as we have seen, are amoral, as in neutral, natural and elemental in their make-up. Again to say, without these forms and forces we could not sin or be righteous; this because they are the means by which good deeds and bad deeds happen.

BUT SURELY, WE MUST BE BADDER THAN THAT?

But what say about verses from Scripture that tell us that we are all *'by nature children of wrath'* (Eph. 2:3)? Or what about King David, who was *'brought forth in iniquity'* (Ps. 51:5)? Surely, these verses indicate that we are all sinful by nature. Let's take a closer look at these two references.

When Adam and Eve sinned, they came under the sentence of *'the Law of sin and of [bodily] death'* (Rom. 8:20), which placed them on the wrong side of God's righteousness. Of this transgression, Paul says that *'the Law brings about wrath'* (Rom. 4:15), which is to say that the nature of our standing in regards to the Law is that of wrath and condemnation. This is why Jesus came to atone for our sins and establish our righteousness before God. When it came to King David, the first thing to note is that he was born in Adam, and thus partook of Adam's iniquity, ie his sin. Also, he had his own list of personal sins, eg adultery and murder, re Bathsheba.

Both of these events had to do with the Law and not some change in human nature. When a robber is caught and tried and sent to jail, his human nature does not undergo a radical change; it remains the same. To make good sense of Scripture, we need to know the difference between the nature of law and human nature itself.

---

desirous

There is a verse in 2 Thess. 1:11 that has kept me believing all these years. There Paul prays for the saints, telling them that *'God will count you worthy of your calling, and fulfill every desire for goodness and the work of faith with power.'* Paul then goes on to say that this human desire for the good must be present in a person's life, *'in order that that the name of our Lord Jesus will be glorified in you, and you in him, according to the grace of our God and the Lord Jesus Christ'* (2 Thess. 1:12).

It is more than evident from these words that if we are unsure of our desires, as in, if we don't trust them, then this will have an adverse effect on our *'work'*, our *'faith'* and our *'power'* (as per vs 11 above). It follows from this that if these three forces – work, faith, power – falter or fail then the *'Lord Jesus [may not be able to] be glorified in you, and you in him'*. To be worthy of your calling, you need to first find and then trust your good desire. The flip side of that, as we have considered, is that if you keep your mind fixed on the instinctual desires of the flesh, making choices on the basis of that desire, then you will sin. Sin, however, is not inevitable, it is always a choice.

AMORAL FORCES IN PLAY

Creatures of pure instinct engage in certain actions that if done by humans would constitute sin. This is to say that it is not so much the activity itself that is the issue for God. Rather, it is the action or deed in its relationship to the creation order – in line with the creation mandate – that constitutes a sin against God or a good deed in the sight of God. As the renowned Dutch theologian G. C. Berkouwer says, *'sin is the act in which we use, or abuse, the reality created by God'* – Studies in Dogmatics, Sin. (Wm. B. Eerdmans Pub. Grand Rapids, Michigan, USA, 1971, reprint 1980), p. 262.

---

strange days have found us

Sadly, theologians down through history have, generally, not affirmed human desire. This, to my mind, has caused lots of problems for Christians trying to make sense of life. By way of one example, have you ever wondered why it is that God gives us a sin nature and then gets angry when we sin? When I first heard this as a new Christian, I thought it was a kind of sick joke; but it wasn't. Our inability to trust in desire has also caused many Christians to remain in an infant-like state in regards to their faith-life. Thankfully, when it comes to the rest of life and work, their desires are not as stunted. As the Christian writer, Dorothy L Sayers said (paraphrased), 'in our everyday work we act as lions, but as soon as we walk through the door of the church, we turn into lambs'.

The church's emphasis these days is more about self-help, positivity and succour for its members. Not many modern church leaders tend to talk about the 'dark-side of the theological moon'. But there it is, at the core of our faith – God's curse, his wrath, our being born spiritually dead and so on. It is as if the church has, in effect, placed this story of wrath and punishment behind closed doors; like some embarrassing relative that you prefer not to mention or, worse, engage. And when it comes to those who put all the bad stuff of life at the devil's cloven hoofs; rather than clearing the air, this approach just compounds our Christian confusion; along with attracting further derision from an increasingly secular culture.

We need to bring God's activities out into the open, and stop being embarrassed at his dealings with humanity. To do this, we need a better theology of sin and the Fall than that posited by the standard historical approach. If we don't do this, our 'embarrassing relative' will continue to turn up and ruin our positive spin on Christendom's wonderful party. To head back to my prior metaphor, re the dark/dank layers of miry clay: if we do not change our way of thinking on this point, this black clammy clay will keep on seeping through the surface of our congregations, and thereby continue to stain and sully our lily-white presentations to the outside world looking on.

underbelly theology

Just in case the reader is thinking at this point that I have over-done this issue of the nature of sin and the Fall, I will present a further example of what troubles me in this matter. To do this, I will be assisted by the *New International Dictionary of New Testament Theology* (Regency, Grand Rapids, Michigan, USA, 1986). In Volume 1, p 457, of this series, a theologian writes about the meaning of the words – *'desire'* and *'lust'*. He says that these two words are often translated in the Gk. as *'epithymia'* – as per the verse in 2 Peter. He then goes on to say, re *'epithymia'*, that the *'noun [form] is found in a neutral or good sense only in Lk. 22:15; Phil. 1:23; 1 Thess. 2:17 and perhaps Rev. 18:14. In all other cases its connotation is bad'*.

This, to my mind, is a useful description of *'desire'/'lust'*, particularly in regards to his mention of the neutral, ie amoral, nature of the body; along with presence of good and bad desires in that body. But what comes next in his description of lust and desire is indeed telling. Suddenly, there is a strange change in the nature of the text, and what this theologian really thinks of human desire rises to the surface – as per his following statements:

- *'Since there is something primitive and instinctive in human desire, Paul maintains that it is recognized as what it really is when the Law speaks to it. This causes desire to become conscious sin'.*

- *'the Spirit replaces desire as the determining power in [a person's] life'.*
- *'[desire] is always lying in wait within a man, so that at the right moment he may yield his will to it and become subject to it'.*
- *'In Johannine writings the origin of desire is traced even further back. It does not originate merely in man but in the 'world' (1 Jn. 2:16), and ultimately [it] comes from the devil'.*

Why on God's good earth did this Bible commentator suddenly decide to jettison his theological neutrality, and from there determine that human desire is ultimately and essentially born of sin and thus, by nature, sullied and sordid. This dark/dank part of Christendom's theology surely needs to be re-examined in the light of a Hebrew day.

theology in need of therapy

This is not just theology we are talking about. It has to do with how people believe and try to live their life and understand God. All those years I spent trying to locate my disenfranchised sin-filled soul, hiding out somewhere in its prison of flesh. What a waste of time that was, and how sad it was that I spent so little time getting to know and work with the instinctual desires of my body of flesh.

Again, I ask the question: in response to human sin, did God crack the very structure of the universe and thereby open up an immense dark chasm in creation and in the human soul – or did he not? In our enquiry thus far into the Genesis 3 account of the Fall, and our consideration of the powerful amoral forces God has put in place, I have not seen any evidence of this dreadful split in the fabric of creation. Indeed, over many years of trying to make sense of the standard account of the Fall, I have come to believe that this horrible rupture in creation and in humanity must only exist in the minds of theologians and church leaders under the sway of Plato's dualistic cosmology. To put it another way, there was no mention of the Fall at the time of the Fall! PS. I will need to keep using the term, *'Fall'*, for my purpose in this book.

How on earth are we Christians going to sustain a story that we can hardly tell our own children, let alone declare it to those outside the Christian camp? I may be wrong; perhaps this life is posited on divine anger and us positioning ourselves for a heaven of the afterlife. Again, the reader will make their choice. But at least there is another choice to be had, one that keeps creation and humanity intact; this so that people can have a chance to grow up and mature within this wonderful and dangerous creation, which, to this day, is still our inheritance in God.

One very useful dividend of this approach to God's creation is that, instead of looking at people coming to you for help and healing, and wondering if they are spiritually dead to God or sinful by nature, you can now engage them in a different way, knowing that you are both, by nature, made in God's own image and likeness; and as such, you are, essentially, just like them!

no big chasm, just same old desires

One last note (for now) on human desire. The *'lust of the flesh and the lust of the eyes and the boastful pride of life'* (1 Jn. 2:16), which, for the most part direct our present-day world systems, is the same bunch of lusts/desires that Eve experienced, pre-Fall, when she *'saw that the tree was good for food, and that it was a delight to the eyes, and that the tree was desirable to make one wise, [and from there] she took from its fruit'* (Gen. 3:6). These desires did not change at the time of the Fall, the reason being that God still has a very important role for them to play in the *'eternal purpose'*.

We humans are not only meant to subdue and steward the entire creation, we are also meant to subdue and care for our very own instinctual body. Paul knew that if he did not overcome the instinctual drives in his body, he would not succeed in subduing and ruling over the vast and wild creation of God. So it is that, if you want to come into your rule over creation, you best start with your own body. Of course, you won't do this perfectly, but you can do it well and good. Let's now engage the last of the four amoral forms and forces – that being *'corruption'*.

08

God Blessed Corruption

In Romans 8:21 we read that the present creation will one day *'be set free from its slavery to corruption'*. This description indicates to us that *'corruption'* is a universal force. The impact and extent of this force is of such as power that it can accomplish the following process: *'you, Lord, in the beginning laid the foundation of the earth, and the heavens are the works of your hands; they will perish, but you remain; and they all will become old like a garment, and like a mantle you will roll them up; like a garment they will also be changed'* (Heb. 1:10-12).

Where do we first read in Scripture about such a force as this? I would say it is in the Genesis 3 account, re Eden and the Fall. As I have said, as soon as Adam and Eve lost access to the Tree of Life they began to physically decay and, in time, physically die. This clearly indicates that universal *'corruption'* must have existed before the Fall. If not, then there would be no need for Adam and Eve to access that Tree of Life. It appears that the fruit of this 'tree' acted as a remedy, enabling the human body to be continually renewed. That is why as soon as the first couple stopped eating the fruit of that tree, their bodies became subject to physical corruption and, ultimately, to physical death.

There are several contenders eligible to do the work of corruption: entropy, leading to disorder via the loss of energy in natural systems (as per the second law of thermodynamics); the sun, which is very energetic, and has the power to prematurely wear out lots of material forms, eg human skin; then there's that strangely wonderful body clock, which gradually winds us all down into old age and ultimate death. I could go on to speak of mildew and maggots, not to mention rust – but enough on that.

ANOTHER ONE OF THOSE PRE-FALL DEATH MARKERS

If animals, fish, birds and micro-organisms did not have access to the Tree of Life, it would mean that, from the beginning, they had a use-by-date. If such is the case, there would have been lots more indicators, pre-Fall, by which Adam and Eve could experience death, and thereby come to understand what God said when he told them, pre-Fall, that *'in the day that you eat from it you will surely die'* (Gen. 2:17).

---

the divine work of corruption

As I have said, sin and righteousness cannot exist by themselves. They need various creation forces designed by God to enable such deeds to happen. All of the forces we have considered are essential to this process, but without *'corruption'* none of these forces could function and do their divine job. So then, when it comes to humans, how does corruption work so as to achieve God's purpose?

For me, the verse that best reveals this truth is Ephesians 4:22. There Paul says that we should *'lay aside the old [Adamic] self, which is being <u>corrupted in accordance with the lusts of deceit</u>'*. What the apostle is saying here is that the measure of *'corruption'* in a person's life will vary *'in accordance'* to the way they steward the instinctual desires of their flesh. To put it another way, the more you misuse or abuse your instinctual nature the greater will be the corruption of your instincts. It follows from this that the more we steward and direct our instinctual nature in line with God's purpose for life, the less will be the impact of universal corruption on our bodily instincts. In the end, of course, corruption will kill us all; hence the need *'to number our days, that we may present to [God] a heart of wisdom'* (Ps. 90:12).

The above information, re instinctual drives, is commonly known, ie lots of people we know (including ourselves!) can find themselves in a place where ongoing bad habits lead to challenges in their body, eg fatigue, depression, illness. I would say that many, if not most of these impacts within the body have their origins in a misuse or abuse of the instinctual desires of the flesh. There are, of course, many other means by which the body can be stressed or weakened, eg poisons, accidents, viruses; this to say that the force of *'corruption'* is not the only player in God's dangerous creation.

weakness works wonders

What is clear here is that God has made the physical creation so that it could be weakened, decayed and subject to physical death and ultimate material dissolution; this so that the impact of human actions could be seen and felt by humans; not to mention the hosts of heavens and God himself. One very big example of corruption's power and purpose is seen in Noah's day. We read in Genesis 6:12 that humans, back then, *'had corrupted their way upon the earth'*. It is a very unusual statement, in the way it's famed. It seems like corruption was once a small river that over time grew into a mighty ocean, doing so in step with human activity. Note that this *'corruption'* makes it *'way upon the earth'*, ie it impacts on the physical earth.

It is also of note that whilst most all of the inhabitants of the earth were subject to corruption, Noah and his clan were not. This clearly indicates that corruption's impact on the human body differs from person to person. Corruption does not itself multiply; rather, the weakening of the body is such that it enables corruption to have a greater impact. As such, the following equations can be postulated – 'the less of the good, the more of corruption' and 'the more of the good, the less the corruption'. To put it in story form – an egg is left in the sun, and another egg is put in the fridge. Two days on, the egg in the sun is on the nose and not fit for human consumption. Five days on, the other egg is fried and eaten, along with mushrooms, to much delight – again to say, both eggs ultimately died.

powerfully blunt diagnostic instrument

This use of corruption by God may seem to some as a rather blunt instrument; but don't be fooled. Yes, we need to consider the Ten Commandments, so as to consider our own and other people's sins. The reality is, however, that it is often difficult for a person to know how to evaluate their own sin; let alone others. Yes, they can acknowledge it, but when it comes to 'measuring' sin there will be many approaches – cultural, psychological, work pressures and so on.

This is why universal corruption is so useful, in that it generates lots more information from the body than that which comes from acts of sin. This, to my mind, is why God designed an amoral elemental force to act as an honest broker; akin to 'Lady Justice', who is often seen outside of courtrooms, representing the idea that justice is (or should be) blind, ie corruption does not see; it just is.

The benefits of this blind corruption and its impact on other amoral forces in the body is that it enables humans to know where they are standing or falling in life. Pain or illness or depression or other physical challenges that emerge from a life which is going against the grain of the good can signal to the person that they should perhaps take stock and change their approach to life. Again, this is a well-worn track for multiplied millions upon millions of people down through the ages; with the modern version being a bit more informed in this regard. As such, it is both a common experience as well as a divine experience.

What we see emerge here is a vast physical creation canvass – animate and inanimate, which holds within and through it the unseen attributes, nature and power of God himself. It is upon this vast canvass of creation that the issues of life and death for every person is played out – as per Deut. 30:19: *'I call heaven and earth to witness against you today, that I have set before you life and death, the blessing and the curse. So choose life in order that you may live, you and your descendants'*.

This divine design of the seen/unseen we have considered establishes the physical frame of the remedial space design of creation – as per, first the natural, then the spiritual. It is from this *'seen'* creation canvass that we can now proceed to fathom more of the *'unseen'* creation forces. These forces are such that they are powerful enough to set the entire creation free from its *'slavery to corruption'* – along with all who seek after life in God – as per Rom. 8:21. The next two chapters (nine and ten) will focus on this universal freedom from physical corruption, from which the unseen inheritance of *'Abba, Father'* will emerge into the hands and hearts of the children.

creation language: see it, feel it, learn it, talk it

In our enquiry thus far we have been able to see (in part) the interaction between the physical forces of the body and God's eternal plan for humanity. This integration between the seen/physical and the unseen/spiritual, I believe, holds the key to (re)generating a form of language that is both old and new; one that will be very useful to those who seek divine meaning and purpose in their work in healthcare and healing. So, what on earth am I talking about?

A person working in healthcare, and who is a Christian, generally has three different forms of language – they being a medical/secular language, their religious/church language and their everyday language. Each language has its own proper place and time in a person's life. It is essential, for example, that medical practitioners and other healthcare workers are able to communicate via a particular form of language or terminology. Also, it is not appropriate for Christians to try and 'push' their religious language into the medical field, as it would only create confusion, or worse. That being said, if that is all there is in regards to the relationship between the medical and the religious, then never the twain shall fully meet; and, as such, the 'seen things' of medicine and the 'unseen things' of the divine will not cross-pollinate as they might otherwise do.

This is why we need to move up a level into what I have called the creation sphere of healthcare and healing. It is from there that we can begin to learn how to speak in tongues that are ancient, but still new. Again to say, this language is generated from the relationships that exists between the seen and unseen, the physical and spiritual, the heavens and earth and, foundationally, between the 'one with' and 'distinct from' design of creation, which, as I have said, has its origins and essence in the Trinity.

It is the life-links between these seen and unseen forms, undergirded by that one with/distinct from design, which is able to create the syntax we need to generate new conversations, and, thereby, new relationships, and from there, more understanding and engagement of that which God has *'hidden since the foundation'* of space and time (Matt. 13:35). It's this language that I needed all those years ago, when working with others in that multi-disciplinary medical practice, trying hard to integrate our Christian beliefs into our practice of healthcare.

language or languish

For those wanting to learn this language of creation, their first steps will involve a good deal of stuttering and stammering. But is that not the case with most new endeavours? If, however, they press on to take hold of this language, the rewards of their work will begin to shine. It is in the light of this Hebraic vision that the language of dualism will begin to fade. From there, verses such as Eph. 3:10, which speak of *'the manifold wisdom of God [that] might now be made known through the church to the rulers and the authorities in the heavenly places'*, will begin to reveal lot's more of their divine and strategic insight; this *'in accordance with the eternal purpose which he [God] carried out in Christ Jesus our Lord'* (ibid vs 11).

The good news is that we are not made to live in Plato's version of the cosmos. Rather, our natural fit aligns with the ancient Hebraic understanding of God's creation. As such, we don't have to strive to take hold of numerous Hebrew doctrines or practices. But rather, drawing from Scripture, we can proceed to engage the actual ground of earth and heavenly skies of which that Scripture speaks. It is in this divinely designed place that our good desires will make their way into lots more of life, work and worship; this in the knowing that we are made for creation and creation is made for us.

Following Paul's advice, re first the natural, then the spiritual – as per 1 Cor. 15:46, we have, in this chapter, mostly focused on the material/physical forms and forces. Now that we have done that, we are eligible to proceed, via apostolic consent, to uncover more of the unseen/spiritual forms and forces that God has made. So then, let's make a move from the *'corruption'* of all physical forms to the human experience of *'futility'*.

09

How to Fill
Disease, Death and Futility

As an introduction to what is to come in this chapter, and the next, I enclose the following divine progression. It is drawn primarily from Paul's teaching in Romans 8, and to my mind it presents us with God's template for human life. I use the word 'template', rather than 'plan', because it does not suggest that the following progression tells us what to do; as in, it does not give us the detail, but rather sets the context within which we can find direction, explore and make choices.

The divine strategy that God put in place for us human beings could be described as one very long game of hide and seek. We read in Scripture that *'It is the glory of God to conceal a matter, but the glory of kings is to search out a matter'* (Prov. 25:2). As such, we who claim to be part of that *'royal priesthood'* (1 Pet. 2:9) need to keep digging deep into the mysteries and wisdom of God. This is your blessing, this is your inheritance; this is life, forevermore. This template or pattern for life, drawn from Romans 8, is as follows:

thorns & thistles + toil & sweat + decay & death (ie corruption) = futility
futility + hope = suffering
suffering + good work = travail
travail = birth
birth = fullness
fullness = inheritance

primal forces of futility

In this chapter I will focus on the first two lines of the template. I begin by exploring the link between the *'corruption'* of all physical forms and the human experience of *'futility'*. The connection between them is found in Romans 8:20-21. There Paul says that *'the creation was subjected to futility, not of its own will, but because of him [God] who subjected it, in hope that the creation itself also will be set free from its slavery to corruption into the freedom of the glory of the children of God'*. It is more than evident from these verses that *'futility'* has a date with destiny; that date being *'corruption'*. Let's look at the chemistry between them.

From the Genesis account we saw how creation responded to humanity's sin by generating *thorns & thistles + toil & sweat*. Also, we noted what happened when Adam and Eve lost access to the Tree of Life – they began their journey into *decay & death*. In chapter three of this book I mentioned that each one of these physical things or forces ensured that no one human (nor humanity in general) could fully access the measure of the unseen 'goods' held in the womb of creation. It is this event, this consequence, which generates the experience of human futility. How so?

Futility is a very human trait. It is not found in dogs, cats or elephants or other creatures of instinct, their needs having most to do with eating, surviving and procreating. Humans, by comparison, are ever restless, wanting more, aspiring, reaching higher. Have you ever noticed that each time you seek to take hold of more or try to move up in life that so often it seems that a veritable litany of that same life is arrayed against you? One might well say that executing a good idea can be the death of you!

Be it in business, government, healthcare or family life, the ability of any process to remain intact and keep working like it should is just not there. Here I am referring more to the relational dynamics of work and family, rather than automated processes, which, of course, have their own measure of mayhem bundled into their technology. Some people who are well-monied can, of course, control life a whole lot more by spending their wealth. Here, however, the markets can intervene, the children can rebel, investments can shatter, and when it is all said, done and dusted, well, you just can't take it with you.

Death is the ultimate futility. We work hard and accumulate lots of things, and then suddenly one day we wake up and find ourselves drawing near to our very own end-of-days. Here pills and medical procedures multiply to fill our time and our bathroom cabinets. But alas, no matter how many preservatives we swallow, still there comes that last hour, minute, second, when *'the silver cord is broken and the golden bowl is crushed, the pitcher by the well is shattered and the wheel at the cistern is crushed'*. This is the time when *'the dust [that is our body] will return to the earth as it was, and the spirit [our breath] will return to God who gave it'* (Eccl. 12:6-7). And what was Solomon's response to all that? '*"Vanity of vanities", says the Preacher, "all is vanity!"'* (ibid vs 8). Note: *'vanity'* is translated from the Hebrew *'hebel'*, which *Strong's* refers to as 'something transitory and unsatisfactory'. As such, this wise-old king of Israel might just as well have said *'futility of futilities... all is futility!'*

I can't get no...

Essentially, our experience of futility arises because we just cannot get hold of the things we want and, if we do get hold of certain of these things, there still seems to be a whole lot more missing! We might call it greedy or grasping, but the fact is that we were made to continually seek for something more in life. In response to these words, one might be tempted to quote the well-known statement of Augustine of Hippo – *'our heart is unquiet until it rests in you [God]'*. This statement is true; but what is also true is that God has established the seen physical forms of life to be the finite containers of his unseen attributes, nature and power. So when we do, as the saying goes, 'find God', rather than resting in that relationship, we are called to get moving all the more into the all things of creation. Relationship with God is never a fixed state. Rather, it is an ever-unfolding experience of relating to and growing in the invisible God (as per Eph. 2:7). As such, every person, Christian or other, has the creation call on their life to seek the unseen goods within the seen things that God has made. Our next step into the progression is *'futility + hope = suffering'*.

live in hope

At the outset of this chapter I quoted Rom. 8:20-21; here, I will focus on vs 20. In that verse Paul said that God subjected the creation *'to futility... in hope'*; this so that creation can ultimately *'be set free from its slavery to corruption'*. I believe that human *'hope'* is that which generates human *'futility'*. How so? Humanity's experience of futility continues, not because the creation has been cursed and is now of little account, but because of that which we continue to hope for in that creation. Logically, if there was little or nothing to be realised in the present creation, there would be little or no desire or effort on either side – creation or humanity – to engage in a meaningful exchange.

It is no wonder that the devil has worked hard and long to take away our hope in the value and purpose of the present creation. But not even this fallen angel can succeed in diminishing or destroying hope in humanity. We humans keep living in hope that we can actually sort out key issues, be they environmental, ethical, technical, political or religious, and that is just the way God designed it to be! Hope is the reason why we keep trying. If there were no hope we would stop and go no further, and futility would cease. This is why God put so much hope in our futility and so much futility in our hope!

I have referred to the impacts of futility, particularly in regards to the physical forces of thorns, toil and death arrayed against us all. Again, what we see here is the way by which the unseen/inner person makes their way through these physical forces, so as to engage the unseen/relational aspect of life. All the way along the line of life these forces of creation are seen, in some way, to be arrayed against us, as what I call 'adversarial allies'. It is this *'futility... in hope'* that generates *suffering* in the inner person. This is not so much about physical pain, even though it can be present or form a part in this suffering. Much more so, however, it has to do with the emotions and desires of the person in the face of challenges and choices.

This suffering, Paul says, holds a big key to our getting hold of God's creation inheritance – as per Rom. 8:17: we are *'heirs of God and fellow heirs with Christ, if indeed we suffer with him – ie Christ.'* I will explore this relationship between suffering and inheritance in detail in the following chapter. For now, let's focus further on Christ's relationship to the creation itself – of which Christ's suffering is, of course, an essential part.

ever-changing contours of creation

Jesus Christ, God-made-man, was not just passing through creation to pay the price for sin, so as to then scoot back to heaven and await the time when the earth and its works would be destroyed, with the forgiven duly plucked out of the mess to join him at his heavenly home. No! Instead, everything he did, including forgiveness of sins, had to do with the Genesis mandate to fill the earth, and thereby fill the heavens (as per Eph. 4:10). This is why all

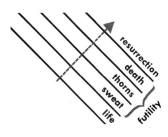

that happened at the time of the Fall leads us into all that happened at the time of Christ's suffering, death, resurrection and ascension. Christ engaged various creation forces such as diseases and demons during his three-and-a-bit years of ministry in Palestine. There is much to glean from his approaches to these forces during his time in a body of flesh. For our purpose here, however, we will take up the account from the onset of Christ's Passion.

First to say, on the day Jesus died he neither became 'sin' itself, nor was he sick, as in filled by disease (as some assert). His presence of mind was strong, his determination stronger, his suffering and sense of going for the joy set before him stronger still. On that day he became *an offering for sin* (Rom. 8:3 and Heb. 10:18). All that he did was *in relation to* sin and all that it had brought to humanity by way of consequences. And what were those consequences? On a physical level this had to do with the growth of thorns and thistles, along with the now diminished capacity of the earth to yield its produce (its fullness), leading to increased sweat and toil in humanity's work. This also included humanity's loss of access to the Tree of Life, which led to the demise and ultimate death of the human body. If we have eyes to see the creation as God sees it, we can begin to fathom the extent to which Christ's Passion encompassed the above-stated forces that generate futility in the inner person. Note the following:

First the thorns: *'Both thorns and thistles it shall grow for you'* (Gen. 3:18). *'And after weaving a crown of thorns, they put it on his head'* (Matt. 27:29). **Then the sweat**: *'By the sweat of your face you shall eat bread'* (Gen. 3:19). *'His sweat became like drops of blood, falling down upon the ground'* (Lk. 22:44). **Then the death**: *'Till you return to the ground, because from it you were taken; for you are dust, and to dust you shall return'* (Gen. 3:19). *'And Jesus, crying out with a loud voice, said, "Father, into thy hands I commit my spirit." And having said this, he breathed his last'* (Lk. 23:46).

all things in Christ

At the time of his suffering and death Christ went into and through the thorns, the sweat and the death. He did this, not to get rid of these forces;

rather, he did this so that he might encompass and thereby fill both the seen experiences and the unseen experiences of futility they generate. By way of example, Christ now fills physical death. As a result of this we now live in a creation in which we are *'always carrying about in the body the dying of Jesus'* (2 Cor. 4:10).

These three powerful 'forces of futility' have a telling and eternal purpose to serve. Now that God the Son made man has filled these forces, he is more than ready and able to direct them in line with his eternal purpose. But there is more! Not only does Christ take the forces and consequences of sin, thorns, sweat and death to himself at the Cross; he also took *'all things'* into himself – all things!

Now that we are able to track Christ's movements in a creational context (as distinct from just the spiritual/religious context) we can begin to see a whole lot more happening on earth and in the heavens. This is particularly so in regards to the thorns, sweat, decay and death that was placed around the fullness of the creation. We can now see Christ coming up and pressing into and through creation's thorns, sweat and death; this with a view to going through into creation's fullness. It is this journey, with its labour of sweat and blood and, ultimately, death, that we must take.

answer to big question

We are now better placed to understand why the children and the rest of creation are made to go through *'slavery to corruption [so as to enter] into the freedom of the glory of the children of God'*? (Rom. 8:21). The reason is that God has subjected the entire creation to the corruption/decay of all physical forms; this in the hope that the 'unseen goods' within creation (ie God's *'invisible attributes, eternal power and divine nature'*) will, over time, be made (indeed compelled) to emerge from the material forms and enter into the heart and stewardship of humans who do the good work and follow truth – as per Col. 1:9-10 and Rom. 2:10.

In chapter five of this book, I referred John 4:24. There Jesus said that *'God is spirit [ie unseen], and those who worship him must worship in spirit and truth'* (Jn. 4:24). Here again, it is evident that our Father God wants us humans to focus on the unseen, so as to progressively engage the *'eternal, immortal, invisible'* (1 Tim. 1:17). Is it not amazing that the entire universe was made so that this movement from the seen to the unseen could happen. Who else but God could dream such a move as this!

PLATO'S TRANSLATORS VS PETER THE APOSTLE

Here follow two versions of creation reality, arising from two translations of the same verse in 2 Peter 3:10, which refer to the last moments of the present universe. The NASB translates this verse as follows: *'the day of the Lord will come like a thief, in which the heavens will pass away with a roar and the elements will be* <u>*destroyed*</u> *with intense heat, and the earth and* <u>*its works will be burned up'*</u>. On the other hand, the Nestlé's Greek Text (Marshall's Interlinear Translation – ILGE) says that *'the heavens... will pass away and the elements burning will be* <u>*dissolved*</u> *and the earth and its works* <u>*will be discovered'*</u>. What then is it to be? All of the universe *'destroyed'* and *'burned up'*, or the physical elements being *'dissolved'* so that the unseen good and/or evil in all of our works might be *'discovered'* (as per 1 Cor. 3:13 – *'the fire itself will test the quality of each man's work'*). Which cosmology will you serve?

---

waiting too long in a queue

All that took place in the incarnation, life, suffering, death, resurrection and ascension of Christ happened *'with a view to an administration [stewardship] suitable to the fullness of the times, that is, the summing up of* <u>*all things in Christ*</u>, *things in the heavens and things upon the earth'* (Eph. 1:10). As such, all that is done in healthcare is now in Christ. This includes the causes of disease, the cures of disease and also death from disease. This view of God the Son coming as man to bring the creation mandate to fulfillment paves the way for new understandings and approaches to healthcare and healing.

As much as we might want to separate the likes of disease and death from our idea of God, we must not. Again to say, did not God himself become flesh, so that he might live, suffer and die for all? As hard as it might sound, we need to know and live in the knowledge that God, not Satan, is at the heart of disease, decay and death. As Paul said, there is *'one God and Father of all things who is over all things and through all things and in all things'* (Eph. 4:6 ILGE).

Humanity is continually lining up against the creation layers of thorns, sweat and death, trying to get through. Now, because of Christ, every person has an opportunity to go through the futility and into the fullness. Now that the Son has come and journeyed into and through creation's womb, the pain of its labour has been intensified. We must learn how to come up to the borders of creation's futility and, instead of stopping and turning away, relegating ourselves again to religious and/or moral containers, we must go through into our inheritance in God.

In regards to those we treat and care for, we need to also know how to engage them in such a way that they too might take their own journey into God. It is the remedial space design of creation that exists to facilitate this journey through creation.

consider this

So then, are we ready to take our inner person (housed in a body so strange and so wonderful) into the decaying forms of the creation, there to engage its futility, with a view to laying hold of the fullness it holds for us? Are we ready to face the forces arrayed against us by this creation reality? To achieve this, we will first have to believe and hope that within and through this vast decay of material forms that the divine good is there to be discovered.

If we do not have this hope, because we have not been given this belief, we will not, intentionally, be able to press up against the thorns, the sweat and the death, and the futility these generate. As such, the journey we were born to make, so as to take hold of our eternal inheritance, will become confused. We surely need to clear the air and end our confusion. In this chapter we have progressed from the *thorns & thistles + toil & sweat + decay & death (ie corruption) = futility* to *futility + hope = suffering*. Four more steps, and one chapter, till we complete what we need to take hold of the remedial space experience. For now, it's time to locate God's birth plan.

10

Contractions in Creation Deliver Fullness

We live in a world of which Christ said, *'nation will rise against nation, and kingdom against kingdom, and in various places there will be famines and earthquakes. But all these things are <u>merely the beginning of birth pangs</u>'* (Matt. 24:7-8). I say we best get with this birth program quickly. For if we don't then we, the church, will continue to experience our precious salt being trodden under foot of all these nations and all these forces!

To take hold of the wisdom of God for creation we will need to become a lot more unsettled. As Christ's body, the church, we should be well and truly 'engaged' by now in this birth process. I fear, however, that at the end of this age many a Christian – be they lay, leader or theolog – will say in regards to a creation they have for the most part overlooked – *'Oops, where did that baby come from?'*

I am well pleased to say that this chapter will be the most strange and wonderful of this book. It is not because I necessarily want it to be strange (or wonderful); rather, it's because Paul the apostle, in Romans 8, made it so! This chapter of the book serves as a culmination and validation of our enquiry, thus far, into the nature, design and strategic purpose of creation. As such, there will be some repetition in what follows in this chapter. Here also I will bring that progression or pattern of life (from chapter nine) to its completion, as per the following last four steps:

suffering + good work = travail
travail = birth

birth = fullness
fullness = inheritance

In the prior chapter we considered why it is that God subjected the entire creation to the decay/corruption of physical forms. The reason is that he wants the unseen things to emerge from there into the heart of humans who dare to believe. We now know a fair bit about this seen/unseen process, but here, in Romans 8, Paul is going to tell us a lot more about it. To do this, he will employ the metaphor of birth. I hasten to add that, for Paul, this birth process is not just a metaphor. The reality is that he believes the physical creation is going to give birth to something magnificent, unseen and eternal.

Such being the case, we need to be very careful how we approach Romans 8. We must ensure that this text is placed in its right cosmological context, ie the Hebraic, and not the Platonic. We need to also consider which version of the Fall will apply to the text – as in, is the post-Fall creation, along with humanity, wholly cursed and corrupted, or not? Another challenge we face is that often theologians tend to consign the strange parts of this Romans text to the end-times and/or age-to-come theological basket – eg *'the whole creation groans and suffers the pains of childbirth'* (Rom. 8:22). This approach disrupts the sense and flow of the Romans 8 narrative, often causing some degree of confusion for the reader.

Theologians are all too often quick to rush past the cursed creation, with all its pain and suffering, and hang on for a heaven of the next life. This 'fast-track' approach reminds me of Adam and Eve and their first sin. Instead of growing up in all of creation like God told them to do, they tried to take a short-cut to heaven; the consequences of which were problematic, to say the least! We need to stay with the creation God has made; this so that the biggest of births will not pass us by. It is *now* that the manifold wisdom of God must be made known, as per Eph. 3:10. Romans 8 is also very focused on the present, from which the future present will, in God's time, arise. So then, let's pitch our tent on the ground of Romans 8 and explore how this cosmic birth will happen.

go get inheritance
We begin at verse 15. It's there we get the good news that we have received *'a spirit of adoption as sons by which we cry out, "Abba! Father!"'*

From there we get even better news; that being that we are *'heirs of God and fellow heirs with Christ, if indeed we suffer with him in order that we may also be glorified with him'* (vs 17). It is evident from these statements that the children are crying out to *'Abba, Father'* for their inheritance. What then is that inheritance?

Before I proceed to the answer that, did you notice something unusual in verse 17? It's the words, *'if indeed we suffer with him'*. It appears from this phrase that the key thing that unlocks the inheritance is *not* holiness or forgiveness or obedience; nor is it about worship, gatherings or leaders, or any other number of good works. Rather, it is our suffering with Christ. Such being the case, we surely need to know the origins and purpose of this unique form of divine and human suffering.

Paul goes on to say that this *'suffering'* is nothing compared to the glory/fruit/fullness it will bring to us (vs 18). At this point, reading about this *'glory'*, one could be tempted to skip straight to heaven; but Paul, at this stage, does not seem interested in that option. What he is focused on is the sight and sound of *'the anxious longing of the creation [that] waits eagerly for the revealing of the sons of God'* (vs 19). The reason for this is that this groaning creation holds with it the children's eternal inheritance.

By way of highlighting this astonishing truth, note the nature of the exchange between the children, *'Abba, Father'*, Christ and the creation (from Rom. 8:15-19). The children cry to the Father for their inheritance, and, in response, he does not immediately answer. Instead, he speaks about the children's suffering with Christ. It is from that mention of suffering that the Father then (via Paul) directs the children to their inheritance, the creation. The inheritance we seek is not found in Plato's version of heaven. Rather, it exists right now, in, through and over all of creation under the third heaven of God's good earth. What we now know is that if we are going to get this inheritance we need to *'suffer with him'* – ie Christ. So then, let's track this suffering and see where it gets us.

It doesn't take long to work out what comes next, re suffering. Paul says in vs 22, *'we know that the whole creation groans and <u>suffers the pains of childbirth</u> together until now'*. Now we are getting closer to the divine action. But there's more: in vs 23 we read that *'not only this [ie creation's groans and suffering in childbirth], but also we ourselves, having the first fruits of the Spirit, groan within ourselves, waiting eagerly for our adoption as sons, the*

redemption of our body' (vs 23). Just as Paul
linked 'suffering' (with Christ) to the children's
inheritance (vs 17), so too, he now anchors this
'suffering' in the creation, which, to this day, is
engaged in 'the pains of childbirth'.

> 'it was fitting for him, for
> whom are all things, and
> through whom are all
> things, in bringing many
> sons to glory, to perfect the
> author of their salvation
> through sufferings'
> Hebrews 2:10

Where there is an impending birth,
there will always be people who care, be they
parents, family, friends, nurses and doctors.
Other visitors to this cosmological birth room
are God the Father, God the Son, God the Spirit, and the children, who are very
excited about this bundle of joy, which is to be fully revealed in God's time.
One of these excitable children is Paul, the doting apostle, who, waiting in
anticipation, says that 'in *hope* we have been saved, but *hope* that is seen is not
hope; for why does one also *hope* for what he sees?' But if we *hope* for what we
do not see, with perseverance *we eagerly expect* it' (Rom. 8:24-25 ILGE). Now
that's what you call a lot of hope placed on this treasure-filled promise!

Note that the child of the womb cannot be fully seen until it emerges.
Not even an ultra-sound can reveal this child, it being but an image of the real
thing. Before we proceed to the birth room of creation, it is essential that we
locate the role that humans play in this birth. I begin this part of our enquiry on
a personal note – as per below:

BEWARE THE END-TIME PLACEBO

Many years ago, I purchased a commentary on Romans, written by Leon
Morris. I don't know which one of my friends stole it, but it disappeared. What I
particularly remember from that commentary was Morris' take on Rom. 8:17-18. He
said (and I am paraphrasing): we need to live with the suffering that exists because of
human sin and God's punishments; but we can take comfort from the fact that one day
this suffering will be no more, this because we will be in heaven.

I read this part of the text again and again, and each time I did, I felt more limp
and useless; having to wait in suffering till God calls time. When I was of a more pagan
ilk, at least I could engage the things of earth and sky. But now, as a Christian, I was told
to detach from these things and forces, and take my daily punishments, with my only
pill being some hope of a heaven of the next life.

The above approach, anchored deep in the psyche of Christendom,
causes believers (generally) to be observers of a fallen and cursed creation;

rather than participants in that creation and its God-given purpose. When it comes to this big birth, we need humans to join in with this process. For this to happen we need to know what God has in view; as in, what is God expecting us to do, so as to bring on this birth? The simple answer is that we need to grow up in all things into him who is the head (Christ) – as per Eph. 4:15. Let's now look at what Romans 8 has to say about us growing up in God.

james and paul, of one accord

In Romans 8:15 we are informed that we *'have received a spirit of adoption as sons by which we cry out to "Abba, Father"'*. One might conclude from this verse that we have now been fully adopted, and thus eligible to receive the Father's inheritance. But when we move on in the text we discover that we are in fact *'waiting eagerly for our adoption as sons'* (vs 22). But how could this be? Have we not been told that *'we are children of God'* (vs 16)? This is where vs 17 helps us by informing us that we are *'heirs of God and fellow heirs with Christ, if indeed we suffer with him'*. Now that's what you call a qualifier, if ever there was one! This verse clearly indicates that just because a person has prayed the sinner's prayer and believes in Christ, it does not mean that they are home and hosed in regards to their adoption and inheritance in God.

In this regard, note again the following two statements: *'[we] have received a spirit of adoption as sons'* (vs 15), and *'we ourselves, having the first fruits of the Spirit'* (vs 23). This indicates to me that God is giving the children what they need at this infant stage, so that they can keep on growing up in all things. The spirit of adoption needs to become the ongoing reality of adoption in a person's life. The Scriptures are replete with verses that speak about this growth and maturity, or lack thereof, eg Matt. 7:22-23, Jas. 2:19-20, 2 Cor. 5:10, Heb. 6:1-2, 1 Cor. 9:27.

This is why we need a lot less observers and a lot more participants in the divine creation plan. Growing up in religion is one thing, but the real thing (with assistance from religion) is about growing up in *'all things'* into God. If we don't do that, and if we don't suffer with Christ, then... well... God is just – it's up to him. I would suggest, however, that we focus a bit less on our congregations and a lot more on our counterpart, the wild and wonderful creation.

a metaphoric summary

I left off in Rom. 8:24-25, with Paul speaking about the hope and expectation of this cosmic birth. It might seem for some that Paul's focus on birth is starting to wane; in that from vs 26 on we don't hear anything more about birth or creation (excepting a reference to *'created thing'* in the final verse of Rom. 8). Instead, Paul, from vs 26 on, begins to talk about the Holy Spirit and intercession and prayers and God making things work for the good, and so on.

No, Paul has not lost the divine plot, re the birth of the unseen goods within creation. Fact is, the apostle has already described what he sees as the process that makes for this cosmic birth. This is revealed in Romans 8:20-21. Let's hear it again: *'the creation was subjected to futility, not willingly, but because of him who subjected it, in hope that the creation itself also will be set free from its slavery to corruption into the freedom of the glory of the children of God'*. Note the prior reference to this birth process in chapter 9 of this book.

We are now well positioned to bring together many of the things and forces we have considered thus far in this book; so as to complete (albeit still in part) our understanding of this biggest of births. Again to say, the following summary will by necessity partake of some repetition. Here follows a succinct description of the process of creation's birth from Paul's perspective.

the womb of creation

God has designed creation so that its seen/physical dimension will continue to push up against the unseen/relational dimension, until such time that God deems that enough of the unseen things have made their way into the hearts of humans who seek for the good in this life. To achieve this, humans have to engage in work in creation. In this work there exists a physical dimension and a relational/spiritual dimension.

When a person is going after the good in their work, they will find themselves pushing up against the physical forces of thorns, sweat, decay and death. This challenge in the work generates relational and spiritual impacts in that labour of work. It also generates the human experience of suffering and futility.

It is in this divine and often fiery furnace of work in creation that human choices are made to live in the flesh or live by the spirit. It is here we decide between the blessing and the curse and, ultimately, between life and death – as per Deut. 30:19. Should one decide for the blessing, they will keep pressing up against the futility forces of suffering and decay, and find themselves in company with Christ, who suffers with them (as per Rom. 8:17). As they continue this good work, they will press up against the unseen womb of creation, thereby generating contractions in that womb.

This divine process will continue until the 'unseen goods' (as per Rom. 1:20) within that womb of creation are finally birthed and given into the hands and hearts of the person who dared to 'good work' God's good earth. Here now finishes the Romans 8 progression; that being the creation's birth, which releases the fullness, which, in turn, releases our inheritance in God. The reader will, of course, decide for themselves whether or not Romans 8 speaks of the release of the spiritual from the natural realm; or not. I myself cannot see a better approach to this most strangely wonderful chapter of Scripture.

release the goods

Just a few more things to cover before we end our Romans 8 enquiry. The reader might be wondering at this stage: 'when does this creation birth take place; is it in this age or in the age to come?' The answer is both. Such is the benefit of a metaphor! In this regard, I mention 'the now, but not yet' expression often found in Scripture. By way of example, in Mark 11:10, Jesus talks about *'the coming kingdom'*, whilst in Luke 17:21, Jesus says that *'kingdom of God is in... our midst'*. This approach is the same that we have considered in regards to the initial *'spirit of adoption'* and the fullness of that adoption.

First to the present age. Each time a person engages in the good work, and thus takes that journey into and through creation, they will release a measure of the goods from its unseen womb. Secondly, in regards to the age to come, this release of the unseen from the seen forms will one day culminate, so much so that God will then decide that *'the heavens... will pass away and the elements burning will be* <u>*dissolved*</u> *and the earth and its works* <u>*will*</u> <u>*be discovered'*</u>. (2 Pet. 3:10 ILGE). It's then that the present creation's *'slavery to corruption'* will have done its work; this by releasing the full measure of the unseen goods held within the physical forms of creation.

> In regards to Christ, appointed for you, *'whom heaven must receive until the period of restoration of all things about which God spoke by the mouth of his holy prophets from ancient time'*
> Acts 3:21

It's from there that all of us will *'appear before the judgement seat of Christ, so that each one may be recompensed for his deeds in the body, according to what he has done, whether good or bad'* (2 Cor. 5:10). For those deemed worthy by God to inherit eternal life, the unseen goods they have gathered in this age will find their way into a redeemed spiritual body. As I have said, if that happens to you, you can be assured of your full adoption, and thus secure in your being an heir of God and fellow heir with Christ. Oh yes, just in case I forgot to mention it: your inheritance will have a whole lot to do with a renewed heaven over a renewed earth – as per Rev. 21:1. Enjoy.

the end begins

It is no wonder that Romans 8 is akin to a theological ride of your life! There is so much to be found in this text that we need to apply to the creation sphere of healthcare and healing. For now, let's complete the Romans 8 road. In regard to this biggest of births we most certainly have to call on the Holy Spirit; the midwife who *'helps our weakness... [the reason being that] we do not know how to pray as we should'* (Rom. 8:26). It is this prayer to Abba Father, this cry, which causes the *'Spirit himself [to] intercede... for us with groanings too deep for words'* (ibid 26). He comes to all who call to him and *'searches the hearts... [and] intercedes for the saints according to the will of God'* (vs 27).

It is here that God's desire meets with good human desire – as per Paul's prayer in 2 Thess. 1:11, *'that the God of us may fulfill every good pleasure of goodness of the work of faith with power'* (ILGE). It is in this place of shared desire – human and divine – that creation joins its own desire, so that together creation's unseen goods can, in good time, be delivered into the heart of humans who dare to follow God the Son. This is the *'will of God'* (vs 27); this is why we have been made to fill the earth by cultivating the ground, the sea and the sky. It's this seen/unseen creation design, in God, that *'we [now] know... causes all things to work together for good to those who love God'* (vs 28). This is why God *'predestined'*, *'called'* and *'justified'* us – all this with a view to our being *'glorified'* in him (vs 30).

I will leave vss 31-37 with the reader, and finish where Paul finished, with this wonderful Hebraic cosmological anthem: *'I am convinced that neither death, nor life, nor angels, nor principalities, nor things present, nor things to come, nor powers, nor height, nor depth, nor any other created thing, shall be able to separate us from the love of God, which is in Christ Jesus our Lord'*

(Rom. 8:37-39). This vast unseen womb of creation, surrounded by thorns, sweat, decay and death, and containing our inheritance, is more than ready to bring to birth. This creation, seen and unseen, is one and the same as the remedial space design we will now explore.

11

Creation's Remedial
Space Design

I begin this chapter with a quote from Jeremiah 29:18. There God says to wayward Israel: *'I will pursue them with the sword, with famine and with pestilence; and I will make them a terror to all the kingdoms of the earth, to be a curse and a horror and a hissing, and a reproach among all the nations where I have driven them'*.

First up, I do confess to having been embarrassed in settings where these kinds of verses are alluded to; particularly if spoken as a taunt by a non-Christian. 'What kind of God is this you serve?' comes their fiery dart; to which my response about the love of God seems rather feeble. For years I took refuge in the belief that these descriptions of events arose because of the 'primitive' understanding of the people of that time. I thought that God was relating to them according to their limited knowledge and superstitious beliefs. Deep down, however, I knew this refuge was just a temporary shelter, one not strong enough to stand the test of time and creation reality.

My other safe-haven from God's distressing words was to tell myself and others that, even though the God of the Old Testament was often angry at people or busy killing them, it was OK because the New Testament God is much more gracious and loving. Thankfully, this unhealthy bi-polarity did not (indeed, could not) last long in my mind. Another option for those who want to protect God's image as a nice person is to outsource most all of the impacts of disease and suffering and death to the devil and his demons. To say, for now, the devil is just not smart enough or strong enough to make pathogens or create death. If he could, then God himself would not be God – and that's just not going to happen!

As a final wrap, re possible make-overs of God's reputation, I note again the plight of Meredith Long (see chapter two). She found it very hard to keep living with the idea that God's wrath and punishment were the reason for most of the suffering, disease and death of those she sought to help and heal. To alleviate her burden she had to shift this curse from the person of God to the creation itself. As a result, for her, creation became *'a terrible enemy'*, one in which *'the natural forces designed by God to express the goodness of his creation [became] the same ones that work towards its destruction'*. This disassociation of God's person and purpose just will not do. We must stay in God. If we don't, then it is going to be very difficult for us to make sense of the remedial space design of God's creation.

see the one, see the all

The righteous Hebrew saw God as the 'first cause' of all things and all events. As dangerous as it might seem to us, they could say that *'If a calamity occurs in a city, has not the Lord done it?'* (Amos 3:6). Exodus 4:11 travels even closer to the bone, with God saying to Moses, *'who has made man's mouth? Or who makes him dumb or deaf, or seeing or blind? Is it not I, the Lord?'*. The Hebrew's first port of call in any negotiation with reality was the person of God. In this regard, note the book of Job, where God allows the devil to test Job via many means, including *'the fire of God [that] fell from heaven'* (Job 1:16), ie not the fire of the devil, but *'the fire of God'*. It was from this kind of stance that the Hebrew could make sense of many more things and forces within creation, including the likes of devils and disease and death.

This approach to life could, of course, tend to fatalism; but for the smart Hebrew (who knew the importance of distinctions) it generated a very proactive approach to life, work and worship. If you start with a pet doctrine or a disease or a devil, you will have very little room to manoeuvre. If, however, you keep looking to the unseen God, you will, from there, be able to go lots more places; yes, at times difficult places, but also deep places, from which old wisdom and new perspectives can emerge.

creation in God, God in creation

This insight into God's relationship to creation causes me to ask the question: when God pursues Israel *'with the sword, with famine and with pestilence'* (Jer. 29:18), is it by virtue of God's power that he instantly makes this kind of judgement happen, or are there creation processes put in place by God from the beginning that can, over time, bring about the above-stated consequences of human action?

I have, of course, weighed this question, so as to encourage 'a yes' to both options. My conviction is, however, that most all of the divine forces that respond to the righteous and the wicked are mediated or enacted within and through the creation itself. This, of course, is no surprise to the readers of this book, who are aware (I hope by now) of the relationship between God's creation and God's person – in that 'one with/distinct from' way.

Yes, of course, in an instant God can (and does) bring on a whirlwind or an earthquake, so as to achieve his will – no problems with that. But there comes a problem when this kind of activity is seen to be God's main form of intervention into humanity and creation. Particularly for those who believe that creation has been sidelined and cursed by God, the tendency is to see God as directing his wrath via the means of a mostly neutral or impassive creation. It's as if God turns up, throws one of his designer thunderbolts into the ground of his now cursed earth, or into the heart of an unsuspecting sinner, and then heads back to his third heaven.

Truth is, however, that our God and father is ever present, *'over all things and through all things and in all things'* (Eph. 4:6 ILGE). Also, as Paul said, God's only Son exists *'before all things, and in him all things [in creation] hold together'* (Col. 1:17). I have mentioned the fear that many have of mixing the seen with the unseen, the natural with the spiritual, and the common with the sacred; again to say, we must grow up and out of this Platonic divide.

The creation is our inheritance; that is why God wants us to search out its very own attributes, nature and power, seen and understood through all that he has made – as

> *'The heavens are telling of the glory of God; and their expanse is declaring the work of his hands. Day to day pours forth speech, and night to night reveals knowledge'*
> Psalm 19:1-2

per Rom. 1:20. God's presence, both within and beyond the creation, ensures that we will never be able to categorically know where the person (or voice) of God starts or stops in regards to a particular action, or where the creation itself starts or stops in regards to its particular actions. It is for this reason that a wise man once said: '*It is the glory of God to conceal a matter, but the glory of kings [and priests, ie us] is to search out a matter'* (Prov. 25:2).

it takes a while for enemy swords to suddenly sharpen

One other good reason why God chooses to most often express himself in and through the creation, is that when things like '*the sword'*, '*famine'* or '*pestilence'* come to town, the average person will not know if it is God who is doing this or if it's just natural forces in play (Note: in Scripture '*the sword'*, when employed by God, refers mostly to the sword of Israel's enemies). Someone like Jeremiah the prophet was able to see the hand of God in these judgements, but most people do not get access to a prophet; particularly a good one! As such, everyday humans need to rely on what is happening in the creation around them; this, so that they can respond relationally to what they think is emerging, in themselves, in other people and in God. After all, it is this creation that we were made to steward and subdue, with a view to our growing up in all things – as per Eph. 4:15. It is for this reason I think that God's use of designer thunderbolts is more the exception than the rule.

Again, I might be wrong; but thankfully, this side of the age to come, I will never quite know! In summary, I would say that the above-stated judgements from Jeremiah most probably emerged from the physical, relational and political environment that was in place around that time; this in a similar (*fractal*) way that the instinctual forces of the human body are able to experience the impact of physical corruption '*in accordance with the lusts of deceits'* (Eph. 4:22) – all this, in line with the God's physical law of cause and effect, and relational/spiritual law of action and consequence.

Note: the word, '*fractal'*, refers to a self-repeating pattern in nature, which is duplicated over and over again from the smallest to the largest iteration, so as to form the entire object – be that a cloud, snowflakes, a tree branch, leaves, skin and so on.

----

live longer; make friends of blessings and curses

I have laboured this issue of God's person and his whereabouts so that as we proceed into the vast creation and its remedial space design we will not have to keep wondering about the location of God's person and presence. All that we have considered thus far in this chapter, re the challenge of staying in God, helps us to now proceed into the big land and open skies of this amazing therapeutic design of life in God.

To lead us in, I again note two key physical forces that work together for the good of God's purpose for humanity – they being the *blessing* and the *curse*. Without them, there would be no remedial space to speak of. We first met with these forces in Genesis. There we noted that, pre-Fall, the ground of earth held the *blessing*; and that after the Fall there came the *curse* within that same ground of earth. As such, the ground now held within it both the blessing and the curse.

To stress the importance of these two natural forces, I again note Moses' words to Israel: *'I call heaven and earth to witness against you today, that I have set before you life and death, the* blessing *and the* curse. *So choose life in order that you may live'*. This verse, in effect, is essentially a description of creation's remedial space design – hence the importance of the blessing and the curse. Let's now expand on the activity of these two physical forces, via assistance from Deuteronomy chapter 28.

TAKE CARE, HERE COMETH THE FORCES OF NATURE
Moses said to Israel that if they obeyed God, then *'all these blessings shall come upon you and overtake you'* (Deut. 28:2) – *'Blessed shall be the offspring of your body and the produce of your ground and the offspring of your beasts, the increase of your herd and the young of your flock'* (ibid vs 4); and, *'The Lord will command the blessing upon you in your barns and in all that you put your hand to, and he will bless you in the land which the Lord your God gives you'* (vs 8) – and from there, on the blessings go!

Moses then said to Israel, that if you do not obey God, then *'all these curses shall come upon you and overtake you'* (Deut. 28:15) – *'The Lord will make the pestilence cling to you until he has consumed you from the land, where you are entering to possess it'* (ibid vs 21); *'The Lord will smite you with consumption and with fever and with inflammation and with fiery heat and with the sword and with blight and with mildew, and they shall pursue you until you perish'* (vs 22); *'The Lord will smite you with the boils of Egypt and with tumours and with the scab and with the itch, from which you cannot be healed'* (vs 27); and, *'The Lord will smite you with madness and with blindness and with bewilderment of heart'* (vs 28) – and on the curses go from there!

These curses are, or course, hard to hear and much harder to bear, but we all know that there are consequences for sin. Be they from the secular or the religious side of town, down through history evil deeds and sinful actions are seen to attract some form of punishment and/or shame. When it comes to God's response to sin and evil, however, it is he who has all power and all privilege to respond to humans in his way. I will speak further on this issue of the curse and the blessing; but for now, it is time to move out and put this remedial space design to work.

one big healing room of life

From our exploration thus far we know that God has designed a creation bounded by and subject to things and forces such as thorns and thistles, unyielding ground, physical decay and bodily death. Within each one of these seen forms and/or forces there exist an unseen counterpart. Together these work to generate relationships between creation and humans, humans and other humans, and humans and God. Let's now place a human being like you or me within this vast creation setting, as per the following graphic:

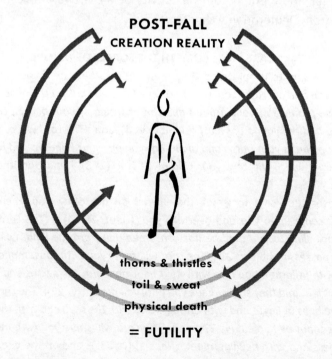

POST-FALL
CREATION REALITY

thorns & thistles
toil & sweat
physical death

= FUTILITY

Let's now look at what creation in God (and God in creation) might do in response to a person who decides to follow a path away from life and into death. Note that the reference to *'death'* in this and other graphics that follow refer to the *'second death'* (Rev. 21:8), as distinct from physical death – see chapter six for more detail on this. For now, following that pattern of action and consequence in response to sin and God's Law, we can picture the following:

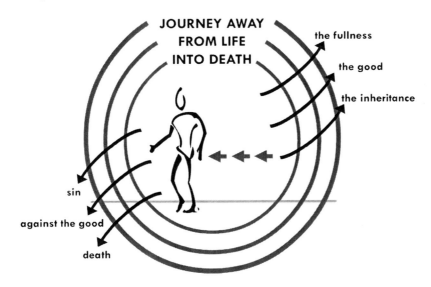

God does not want any person to perish, and, as such, he has designed a creation in which those who are going after the *'second death'* (instead of life) will be challenged in regards to the course they are taking. What then might God do in response to such a movement away from life and into death? From our reading of Deuteronomy we get a sense of the many and varied options that he has in his creation store.

I have referred to the thorns and forces of the curse and the way in which they arise in and from the ground of earth. This ground, as we know, also holds multiplied trillions of bacteria and viruses, which daily seek to engage the human body. Let's now see what might follow from a dispatch of 'pestilent pathogens' into the body of a person who is going the wrong way in life. As one rapper once said – *'oops, there goes gravity'*.

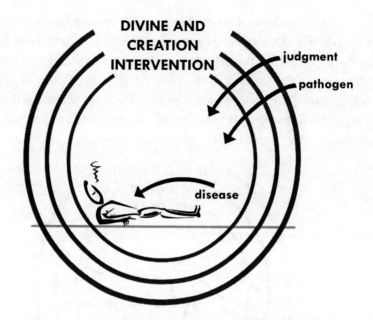

One of the first things often noticed when a disease takes hold of a person is the weakening effect it has on the body. Paul speaks of the sins of certain saints, saying that *'for this reason [ie their sin] many among you are weak and sick'* (1 Cor. 11:30). Illness diminishes the power of human instincts, be that in relation to appetite, sexual desire or one's self-confidence. This 'weakening' of the flesh causes a person to become more responsive to the forces that generate *'futility... in hope'* – as per our consideration in chapter nine. What we see here is illness as a form of intervention, which serves to slow down or even stop a person in their journey away from life in God.

People who are sick and sane will most often seek relief for their pain and suffering. A visit to a pharmacist or a medical doctor or other health carer will often result in some kind of initial relief, along with, in many cases, a preliminary understanding of the illness. Particularly in the case of those who are overcome by the initial intensity of their disease, these interventions help them to distinguish more clearly between themselves and the disease. Added to this is the presence of those who come to comfort and/or pray and/ or otherwise attend to the needs of the sick person. All this serves to enlarge the relational context within which the sick person engages with their illness.

It is this 'common' process that enables the person in view to not only rest, but also to contemplate their state of being and/or way of life. The level of this reflection will, of course, depend on the person's circumstances in mind and body. In a general sense, however, what we see emerging here is a process by which the remedial space opens up, so at to establish a larger setting in which reflection and conversations can begin to take place, as per the following:

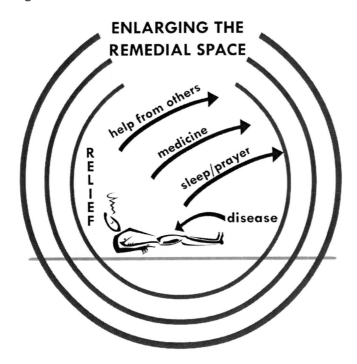

ENLARGING THE REMEDIAL SPACE

RELIEF

help from others

medicine

sleep/prayer

disease

It is this remedial space, working within and through the seen and unseen things and forms of creation, which enables a person to do business with life in God. This amazing space, triggered in this instance by infection, held open by suffering and weakness, and enlarged by pain relief and other medications, along with care from others, is a vessel most ready to serve God's purpose for humanity. It is within this remedial space design of creation that each person is given an opportunity to respond to their way of life, as it relates to others, to creation and, ultimately, to God, as per the following:

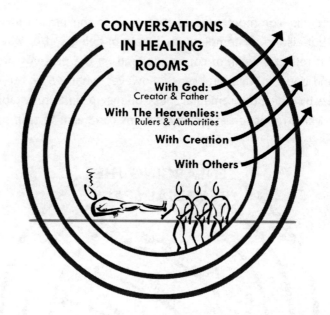

don't side step the dance

What we see in this remedial space design is essentially therapeutic and, thus, restorative in its divine intent. In response to this, however, many believers will still be left wondering why God has to respond to sin in such a primitive, drastic and oh so visceral way – as per Deut. 28. Yes, the idea that illness is part of God's response to human sin is acceptable to most Christians. But really, I hear someone say: 'when it comes to assimilating the curses of Deuteronomy 28 into the remedial space design, for me and most people it's a curse too far!'

In response to that, I could try and ease the reader's burden by saying that at the time Deuteronomy was written Moses was trying to get the tribes ready to inhabit the land of Canaan. And as such, he had to scare the wits out of all of them so as to get their attention. Added to this, I could say that the culture of ancient times was different to our own sophisticated and more caring culture; or I could go for that split between the Old Covenant God and the New Covenant Son of God. From there, I could keep going; whittling down the hard words of Moses until they faded like watermarks on Old Testament paper. But all this would do little justice to God's person and purpose – or for you and me.

Soften the blows of Deuteronomy if you need to; but do not extinguish in your mind the divine intent of these forces of nature. On this list are *'pestilence'*, *'tumours'*, *'madness'* and *'bewilderment of heart'*, all made and held by God, for his eternal purpose. Again, we need to stay in God, so as to learn why he sends us things and forces such as these. The first step into this learning and discovery is to listen to Scriptures that speak of God's intent – as per: *'It is I [God] who put to death and give life. I have wounded and it is I who heal'* (Deut. 32:39). And from the prophet Hosea, *'Come, let us return to the Lord; for he has torn us, but he will heal us; he has wounded us, but he will bandage us'* (Hos. 6:1). We must take hold of God's therapeutic intent for humankind. I would go so far as to say that it holds the key to unlocking the creation mandate.

questioning the deuteronomy

At this stage of our inquiry into the remedial space design there will, of course, be many questions to answer – such as, 'what about people who have not made bad choices, but still get horrible diseases?', or 'what about those who do not have the ability to make right choices?'; or 'God's use of pathogens in this depiction seems to me to be a very blunt instrument by which to measure a person's moral status'. I am sure that readers will add many more questions.

What I have presented here is simply a template by which we might begin to engage in further conversation and consideration of God's plan for humans; this to say that I do not plan to solve the world's problems via a few graphics! These verses about the curses we have considered do not constitute a medical model. However, they can, I believe, speak to us (over time) about the nature of disease, decay and death. Truth is, to this day most humans seek for some kind of meaning in their experience of disease and death. As such, we who believe need to ensure that this meaning does not itself die a secular death.

I (Thwaites) was giving a one-day work-shop for healthcare workers, during which I asked the following question of a doctor who worked in palliative care: 'Would you rather die of a heart attack or from cancer?' He was seated when I asked him that question and on hearing it his head slumped to the table and remained that way for many long seconds. Finally he lifted up his eyes, which were blue and deepened with the reality of many deaths, particularly from cancer, and he said: 'I would rather die from cancer, because with cancer you get time to tell your truth'.

For me, when I compare the Deuteronomy list of curses to the incredible sophistication of modern-day medicine, I am still somewhat embarrassed; particularly in the company of those of a secular persuasion. But it is only for a little while. After that my blushing fades and I remind myself that, as amazing as modern-day healthcare is, it is still just one facet of life.

It is from this 'Deuteronomy template' of the remedial space design that we now dig deeper, so as to find more divine wisdom – *'hidden from the foundation [of all created things]'* (Matt. 13:35 ILGE). To do this, we will pay a visit to Job. He was a Hebrew fellow, who is said to have lived at the time of the Judges, a few hundred years before the first monarch was installed in Israel. Job was a righteous man, and because of that he was afflicted by disease; and that with God's express permission. How strange and hard-to-bear is that!

Paul said in Romans 8 that if we are to get hold of our inheritance in creation, we will have to *'suffer with him'* (Christ). If this suffering was good for Paul and it's good for Job, then surely it must be good for us. Such being the case, let's now study the 'Job template' – so as to complete the circle of creation's remedial space design.

12

Remedial Space
Comes Full Circle

The book of Job contains yet another disconcerting moment for believers of a Judaeo-Christian persuasion. Here God contends with the devil to see who is right in regards to Job's character. The words we read in this book of the Bible are stark, shocking and hard to bear – as per, *'Satan answered the Lord and said, "Skin for skin! Yes, all that a man has he will give for his life. However, put forth thy hand, now, and touch his bone and his flesh; he will curse thee to thy face." So the Lord said to Satan, "Behold, he is in your power, only spare his life"'* (Job 2:4-6). The results that followed from this deal are enough to make a hard-edged theolog wince!

Here is Job, living in a fallen creation, constrained by thorns and toiling away. He seems to be making a good job of it. He knows that even though creation has been somewhat altered as a result of the Fall, it is still the creation of God. Job was one of those who saw the unseen and thus sought out *'the goodness of the Lord In the land of the living'* (Ps. 27:13). He was definitely one of those people who *'by perseverance in doing good [sought] for glory and honour and immortality, eternal life'* (Rom. 2:7). Or was he? This was the issue in question.

To determine the answer, a select group of creation forces entered into Job's spacious compound. These included *'the fire of God from heaven'* (Job 1:16), three marauding bands of Chaldeans (ibid 1:17), *'a great wind from across the wilderness'* (1:19) and, on the second round, a bunch of *'sore boils from the sole of [Job's] foot to the crown of his head'* (2:7). The *'very great'* pain that Job felt from these intruders stopped him in his tracks and opened up Western history's most well-known remedial space experience. It was within this divinely-designed creation space that conversations both old and new could unfold.

spatial character analysis

In every remedial space there are many players and forces involved. The focus is most often on one person. However, as they say, no person is an island. God, the practitioner, family, friends, pathogens, enemies, instincts, angels and devils, indeed, any one or more of all *'things in the heavens [as well as] things upon the earth'* (Eph. 1:10) could possibly enter into one of creation's healing rooms. (Note: the phrase, 'creation's healing rooms' is the same thing as the remedial space design; its distinction being that it refers more so to the individual's remedial space experience – in a fractal way.)

In the background of Job's trials stood God and the devil, both of whom were instrumental in triggering his remedial space experience. In the foreground there are five main players, Job's wife, the three so-called comforters, and near the end of the experience, a young man, Elihu, who put his penny's worth into the mix. Job's wife tried to shut down the remedial space encounter, by advising Job that he should *'Curse God and die!'* (Job 2:9). Yes, physical death was an option for Job, but in his estimation, for now, life was worth the living.

The problem all four men had with Job was that he believed that *'he was righteous in his own eyes'* (ibid 32:1) and thereby had *'justified himself before God'* (32:2). It was, however, obvious to at least three of Job's friends that he had sinned against God's Law. The reason they were so confident in their moral assessment was that Job's hair follicles had turned into inflamed pus-filled lumps from *'the sole of his foot to the crown of his head'* (2:7); not to mention all of his other recent misfortunes.

Deuteronomy and the old school tie

The three comforters (minus Elihu for now) had, is seems, been well trained in the school of Deuteronomy. We have read about this school of divine thought, particularly in regards to its focus on the blessings and the curses. There Job's three companions learned the following equation: sin = divine judgement = disease +/– calamity +/– madness +/– death. Along with this, of course, came the blessing, which was, in effect, the opposite of the above equation. So entrenched was this doctrine of curse and blessing in the Law of

Moses that it became the primary means of assessing peoples' righteousness or wickedness.

But here comes Job, with his boils and tragic misfortunes, and dares to take on this fundamental doctrine of sin and divine punishment. Job got sick and sad, but he didn't think he was sinful. This, to his comforters, was a kind of heresy. Thirty long chapters, give or take a verse or two, were given to this tussle between Job and his three uncomforting friends – and none of them got over it. By the end of chapter 31 Job was well and truly worn out; so much so that the writer of Job's account said: *'The words of Job are ended'*.

But just as Job was about to close his eyes – in the hope, perhaps, that when he opened them his three friends would not be there – the young man, Elihu, took his chance to give Job some advice. His two main bullet points were these: God chastens people beforehand so that they will not enter into sin later on (this is similar to Hebrews 12:5-13); and, God is so far beyond us and so amazing that anything he does is for the good, be it for the boils or the spoils (ie of war). It's of note here that this young man did not entirely beat to the old-school Deuteronomy drum. This, I would say, is why, when God finally turned up, he did not ask Elihu to offer a sin offering; as distinct from Job's three friends who did. It was towards the end of Elihu's five-chapter speech (chapters 32-37 end) that he began to wax lyrical about God's amazing creation, so much so that he started to slip into the very same story that God was about to tell. Maybe that's why God suddenly turned up, via a whirlwind, and finally began to talk. And what a story God had to tell!

job's push into creation

If I was Job, I would be extremely interested in asking God the question – 'why, why, why, and where were you when I wanted you?' But there was no time for Job to even frame a question like this; the reason being that God just kept on talking and talking without stop for four chapters. In God's introduction to these chapters, there was no mention of why all these terrible things happened to Job, no mention of the devil's wager and no mention of Job's righteous standing, or otherwise. All God wanted to do was to talk about the wonderful creation he had made; this along with (shall I say) somewhat of a sting in certain of his words – as per, *'Where were you when I laid the foundation of the earth? Tell me, if you have understanding, who sets its measurement, since you know?... Or who laid its cornerstone when the morning stars sang together and all the sons of God shouted for joy?'* – and so on, from chapter 38 to end of 41.

When God finally finished, Job had very little to say, except to say: *'I know that Thou canst do all things... I have declared that which I did not understand, things too wonderful for me, which I did not know. Hear, now, and I will speak; I will ask you [God], and you instruct me. I have heard of you by the hearing of the ear; but now my eye sees you. Therefore I retract, and I repent in dust and ashes'* (42:3-6). From there, God does some divine housekeeping, telling the three (now apparently) unwise men that they *'have not spoken of me [God] what is right as my servant Job has'* (42:7) – hence their sin offering. From there, Job gets a twofold increase of all that he had lost. After that he lived 140 years and then died, *'an old man and full of days'* (42:17).

suffering in forward motion

There is, of course, lot's to tell from this tale of Job and his sufferings and restoration. The first thing to say is that Job has helped us subvert the 'Deuteronomy template'; but in a good way; as in, not to extinguish or discount it, but, rather, to complete it. Thanks to Job, no longer could it be said that the Scriptures endorse the idea or doctrine that suffering and/or misfortune are always the result of sin. Yes, it can be a result of sin, but again to say, we will never be able to know if it is or is it not.

This is why we need to rely less on moral judgements in our evaluations of ourselves and others, and more on the creation processes that God has put in place. By saying this, I do not mean that humans should not *'have their senses trained to discern good and evil'* – they should (Heb. 5:14); but it takes more than just individual discernment to decide, re the issue of good and evil. As I have said, it is the creation forces of the blessing and the curse that best *prove* the nature and character of our bad and good deeds.

With encouragement from God's creation speech, Job was also able to realise that there is something even more important than justifying one's self before God; and that was God's call on Job's life to fulfil the Genesis mandate, as per Gen. 1:28 and Ps. 8 and Eph. 1:23. This progression from one's righteous standing to one's standing in creation is alluded to in Hebrews 6:1-3. There the writer says that, *'leaving the elementary teaching about the Christ, let us press on to maturity, not laying again a foundation of repentance from dead works and of faith toward God... and eternal judgement. And this we will do, if God permits'*. It was Job who made his move (with a fair bit of push and shove from God) to go past the elemental law and begin to engage a whole lot more of his creation inheritance in God. This increased standing in creation and in God is evident from the last seven verses of the book of Job.

This 'forward movement' (via the remedial space) into more of creation, and thus more of God, is endorsed by the great physician himself. In response to seeing a man born blind, the disciples said to Jesus, *'Rabbi, who sinned, this man or his parents, that he should be born blind?'* (The elementary school of Deuteronomy was still very much the dominant doctrine at that time). In response to his disciples, Jesus did not even countenance the question. Instead, he told them that *'it was neither that this man sinned, nor his parents; but it was in order that the works of God might be displayed in him'* (John 9:2-3). Jesus was not ruling out sin, be that in the man born blind or in the disciples! What he was saying is that this person's issue is not so much focused on where he came from, but rather where he is going to – that being (hopefully) towards the full measure of the good – ie *'the fullness'*. This aligns with the last graphic in the prior chapter, with one exception; that being to replace the word 'judgement' with 'intervention'.

We need to move beyond our elementary doctrines, not because they are no longer useful or valid, but, rather, so that we can achieve their purpose, which is to establish foundations upon which growth and maturity in creation can proceed. This kind of growth cannot take place in church meetings. Yes, it can be rehearsed in the gathering, but not for too long, lest we mistake the rehearsal for the reality. Our mandate to fill all things in all dimensions can only happen in and through our work in God's good creation. It is there that our inheritance is crying out to us, waiting for us and wanting us to engage the good work, so as to release the unseen from the seen.

one more run thru curse and blessing

To say, yet again, it being such an essential truth: the blessings and the curses are always found together in the ground of creation and, thus, they are also found in the human body. When a person goes against the grain of God's good creation, the curse is able to rise from the ground, so as to become their most efficacious remedy. Should they begin to respond, by turning from death to life, then this curse will start to be overtaken by the blessing. And for those who seek for the good in life (like Job), they too will embrace the thorns, sweat, decay and bodily death, born of that same curse – so that it might serve as their strong-suffering tonic, along with, or course, that sweet nectar of the blessing, felt from ground to scented sky.

The experience of most healthcare practitioners is that many people who present for assessment are not sick with 'diseases' we can readily identify and treat. Rather, they are unwell because of relationship and social problems; often compounded by bad choices and poor support networks and coping strategies. Modern medicine, however, often has little or no time, or has no framework to acknowledge this human part of health and healing. Many of these people, as we know, become more susceptible to both disease and chronic illness because of their inner problems and lack of support. Hence the need to make space for those conversations in the healing rooms.

Nicola Cooper, Medical Doctor, UK

———————————

This creation template of the remedial space is not the only one on offer. But that being said, it is a very big player in God's eternal plan for humans. Its borders are established from the third heaven down to and around the ground of planet earth. Its composition is made up of seen forms (which are temporal by nature), within which exist the unseen forms (which are eternal by nature). Most all of this action in creation is found first in the natural realm. From there, and only there, can the spiritual and relational dimensions within the physical creation do their thing. It is within the ground of earth, along with the rest of the physical universe, that forces such as corruption and decay and death emerge to do business with both the 'outer man' and the 'inner man'. There are, of course, more things and forces that we have considered throughout this book that I did not mention above. But in summary to say: it is this remedial space design that leads all these things and forces we have considered into a most sublime and divine cosmological dance!

thanks for the boils

The remedial space experience is not limited to the sphere of healthcare. Rather, it is part of every facet of life, work and relationship. That being said, those who are involved in healing professions, by virtue of their work, will engage this remedial space more often than those in other spheres of work. Such being the case, healthcare workers do have an important part to play in peoples' remedial space experience. We will look at the nature of this stewardship in chapter thirteen.

Our more intense encounters with this part of God's divine design can be brought on by Chaldean armies, wind from across the wilderness, the loss of assets, the birth of a child, financial windfalls or job promotions, as well as illnesses. It is as we age and begin to enter into our time of dying that this remedial space will increasingly respond to us. As such, we need to get to know this gift of God sooner, rather than later; so that we might work with this divine design and not against it.

As a sign off on this chapter I offer the following thoughts: I do not believe that disease has a voice of itself; but as a force to be reckoned with, it can certainly help a person find their voice and speak their truth. Is every disease a result of personal sin? No. Does every disease carry a measure of reality, a measure of truth-telling in its delivery? My sense is to say a careful yes to that. Can disease be used by God to bring us into more of life and maturity? I would definitely say a yes to that.

To this I add two quotes from a seminal practitioner of medicine who lived in ancient times. His name, Hippocrates (circa 460BC-370BC). Some Christians might wonder if he was kosher; he having experimented with many things and forces within creation. But I would say, in line with his words below, that he searched for truth, and for the good of those he sought to help and heal – as per the following:

'A wise man should consider that health is the greatest of human blessings, and learn how by his own thought to derive benefit from his illnesses.'
&
'It's far more important to know what person the disease has than what disease the person has.'

Selah!

13

Conversations in the Healing Rooms of Creation

One day we each will die. For you, the reader, it could be in a year or ten or thirty or more. The fact is that no pill, procedure or practitioner will ultimately stop this death from happening. In regards to your impending death, what will you make of you; what will others make of you; and what will your maker make of you?

Those who believe in the eternal one know that this third question speaks to our ultimate epitaph. One day, God will give a speech about your life, and he will tell you your real story. It's scary, I know; but it is also amazing. Such being the case, the story of your life is of eternal importance to you. Thankfully, our story is not predestined (as some say). It is formed and unfolds as we move into and through our lives – with all its bad, embarrassing days, and its good, exultant ones. Your story, along with all others, will be written down in the *'deeds in the body'* (2 Cor. 5:10), which you have carried through the days of your life.

Historically, many cultures have seen the story of one's disease as being important, if not more important than the disease itself. In many instances they saw the story as holding the keys to the cure of the person. This, of course, is a practice that has sometimes worked for good and sometimes not for good. Again, however, it indicates humanity's need to search for meaning and purpose in illness and in death. Not only does the story of a person's life hold immense importance to them; it also impacts on those who influence and engage with that person.

tell your story

The experiences of creation's remedial space that we have throughout our lives most certainly form a large part of our story in God; hence the need for us to consider learning how we might engage with this divine design. This, of course, is particularly relevant for those who believe in God and also work in healthcare and healing professions

My intent in this chapter is to consider how Christians might engage this remedial space design within the context of their work. In saying this, it might appear that I am edging my way into some kind of healthcare model. But such is not the case. Rather, my intent is to even further distinguish between the story (or narrative) of modern medicine and the story of every person in God. To begin this enquiry, I note the following account of one person's experience of modern-day medicine.

In the medical system the practitioner's beliefs and emotions are seen as irrelevant to the process of medical treatment. Instead of looking into the bigger picture of what might be happening, you are pressured to comply with just those things that the system requires or demands. The effect of this is to make you as a person feel like you are removed from the work you do.

This approach is presented as something that creates safety and security, and this is, of course, one of the benefits or reasons for that approach. But, because it does not allow you, the person, to engage those you work for in a more humane manner, such an approach doesn't really work well. Instead it isolates you. Sometimes I have woken up in the morning and wondered why I was coming to work.

Cate Hayes, Medical Doctor, Australia

---

subject to object

Not only Cate Hayes, but also the many people who come to her for help and healing, seem to be missing something of value. Thus the need to explore that interface between seen/objectivity and unseen/subjectivity. To do this we will need assistance from that 'one with/distinct from' design, which, as I have said, has its origins in the Trinity. I begin with the objective side of this often strained relationship between seen and unseen.

The fact that modern-day medical science is focused on physical forms, rather than metaphysical or religious considerations, makes it a very useful and necessary discipline in today's multi-ethnic societies. Modern-day healthcare exists because of a societal consensus; a primary part of which is government. Such being the case, healthcare professions and institutions ultimately come under the rule and authority of the state. This ensures that no one healthcare practitioner will be able to change the rules to suit their own religious beliefs, and if they do, they will be subject to censure by their rulers and authorities.

It would seem by this reckoning that Christians trying to introduce the idea of the remedial space design into their work in healthcare will be met by their peers and/or their bosses with a no-show. It's here, however, that the unseen/relational (ie the subjective) emerges to show us a better way! This way ahead is led, yet again, by the apostle Paul, who says in Titus 3:1 that we have *'to be subject to rulers, to authorities, to be obedient, [so as] to be ready for every good deed'*.

Yes, this verse does seem rather tame, but don't be fooled. In effect, what Paul is saying here is that if you do the right thing by the established rulers and authorities, then you can go for it in regards to getting on with doing good things in your work in healthcare and healing; this in line with that blessed societal consensus I referred to. This seemingly small part of the healthcare landscape holds the key to a whole lot of unseen/relational treasures – one of which goes by the name 'remedial space'. Here follows a graphical representation of the distinctions I will be considering in this chapter.

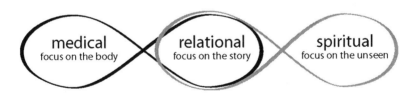

who has what time it is

Before I proceed to map this thin but deep slice of modern-day medical practice, I need to have a conversation with the doctor and the nurse, along with other believers in God who are in that healthcare mix. I have heard their strings of stress, singing the healthcare song that goes by the name – *'the impossible dream'*. As in, I have heard the doctor and the nurse tell me that they are very busy, often tired, and at times worn out. And as such, how on earth (they politely say) is it possible for us to make room for this 'remedial space thing'.

I mean, it sounds alright (said the nurse), but who has the time; and will this be at the expense of patient care? To which the busy doctor added:

what are the risks involved, in regards to possibly putting religious pressure on clients; and what of possible litigation if something goes wrong from this remedial space approach? Perhaps (they politely say) we could hand this kind of thing over to hospital chaplains or local pastors or, maybe, Christian therapists – or all of these. My response to that is, yes, these and other in-kind professions will most certainly be eligible for this task. But to my mind, if we minus the medical, there will be a vast gap in our population who will miss the measure of this remedial space action.

In regards to the concerns of the nurse, doctor and others, my initial response is to say that from the time they were both born they have been immersed in this remedial space design – as are all the people they seek to help and heal. This is to say that the remedial space design is inherent in humanity and in the rest of creation; rather, than it being an add-on after the fact. As such, this is about the possibility of enlarging the scope of our present work, in line with God's purpose. To put it another way, this is a case of *'whoever has, to him more shall be given'* (Luke 8:18).

One of the reasons why the doctor's concerns need not be realised is that, in what I am considering, there is no requirement for any direct spoken religious activity to take place between the practitioner and the patient. I know this might sound strange, particularly seeing this chapter is called 'Conversations in the Healing Rooms of Creation', but my approach to this is to follow Christ; this by being *'wise as serpents, and harmless as doves'* (Matt. 10:16 AV). I will, of course, expand on this somewhat meek approach as we continue. For now, let's get back to that thin/deep/relational space I referred to in Titus 3:1, re, 'go the good work'.

to pray or not to say

Again to say, we need to distinguish between the medical, which is anchored in human rule and authority, and the relational and spiritual aspects that exist in modern-day healthcare practice. Note: as I have said, the relational and the spiritual are one and the same. But for most people this will be hard to understand; hence the three – medical, relational and spiritual – in the above diagram. Let's now briefly look at how we might negotiate between the medical and the relational/spiritual, via some examples.

A Christian fellowship in a hospital has a lunchtime prayer meeting in the chapel, during which they pray for each other and, in a general manner, pray for staff and clients – no names please. Some might consider first names, but I think that's a problem. Apart from the issue of names, I would say that this activity complies with rule and authority. What about a hospital chaplain with a team of lay-workers, who encourage and pray with patients who request such activity? No problems there, in regards to being *'obedient, [and thus]... ready for every good deed'*.

What if a client is asked about a spiritual or religious issue they are challenged with? Of course, the practitioner can respond to this, even if by referring to their faith, but don't get carried away. Keep in step with your client, and don't take opportunity to witness for your faith. What if a Christian who works in healthcare speaks out against issues such as abortion and euthanasia? In our current healthcare system you cannot, when at work, speak out on these issues. At home or, say, at a Christian convention, a person is free to do so. The rulers and authorities might hear about this conference, and thus might frown upon the individual in question. But they have no right to censure this person.

Some believers pray for reconciliation between healthcare and Christianity. Others pray in relation to past and present sins of the medical profession, so as to cleanse or redeem healthcare – no problem, as long as this happens off-line from the work place. And when it comes to a silent prayer at work for a patient or a colleague or a challenging issue, *'against such things there is no law'* (Gal. 5:23).

mixing powers

In the multi-disciplinary practice I referred to in the author's preface, a few doctors would ask their clients if they would like to be prayed for at the end the session. It was known that the practice was populated by Christians, and, as such, a number of Christians were keen to be prayed for by their doctor. This prayer was offered to many, Christian or not. Of course, in this activity, the doctors were careful and discerning.

At first I thought this was a good thing, but a few years into the practice I was not so sure. What concerned me was that the doctors were drawing on the authority of their profession and associating that authority with their religion. This, to me, was not in line with the consensus of their profession; hence the challenge to this activity, in regards to the rulers and authorities established by God.

As team leader I did not feel to stop this practice, one of the reasons being that I was not in charge of the doctor's specific practice. Also, quite a few people benefited from the prayer. Still, however, for me this became an operational and strategic theological issue pertaining to God's intent, as per Rom. 13:1. I will go into more detail on the issue of rule and authority in the following two chapters. Again, this is not a detailed summary of what Christians working in healthcare should do or not do. Rather, it is intended to assist them to negotiate the different facets of their work – so as to keep them moving within the divine streams of human work, and not be compromised. So then, what comes next?

oblique divine strategy

I think what's next is the Genesis mandate. After all, it is this divine plan that takes into account all the things and forces that make for the seen/medical, the unseen/relational and the unseen/spiritual. One of the things about that vast creation mandate to fill the earth is that in its operations it is often not very direct; this, say, in comparison to evangelising or discipleship or preaching in and from the gathered church setting.

In this regard, note again that verse from Matt. 5:16, where Jesus said: *'let your light shine before men in such a way that they may see your good works, and [thereby] glorify your Father who is in heaven'*. Again to say, this doesn't seem to be a very direct approach to achieving God's plan for humans. I would say the reason for this is that God's is very interested in the relational dimension of life, and less interested in process – as in, say, seven steps to grow a big gathered church.

What this verse from Matthew suggests to me is that if we align with God's plan for creation then our work will impact for the good on the people we serve in healthcare. To follow this somewhat 'roundabout' relational strategy, we will need to trust God's creation to do its work within us and with others. In our enquiry in this book, we have been able to take hold of lots of useful things and forces that God has made – for just such a purpose as this. Let's now proceed to apply some of this 'roundabout' strategy to an everyday consulting room.

the common divine

No matter who a person is – a saint, an agnostic, a pagan or atheist, each will carry their world-view in some way into their work; and so should you! For those who seek after God, there are many divine things on offer in hospitals and consulting rooms; such as: *'if two of you [ie practitioner and patient] agree on earth about anything that they may ask, it shall be done for them by my Father who is in heaven'*. And not only that, but also *'where two or three have gathered together in my name, there... [God is] in their midst'* (Matt. 18:19-20). Now that's a good thing!

All well and good (I hear some say), but tell me, how can you have an agreement if the other party, ie the patient, does not have a clue about what you're thinking? By way of an indication, re this unspoken approach, I mention the Holy Spirit, who, when joining the cry of creation to the desire of humanity, is said to have interceded for us *'with groanings too deep for words'* (Rom. 8:26); hence the divine precedent. Here follows a more down to earth example of this kind of exchange from Dr Nicola Cooper, UK. Note, in particular, the second paragraph of her extract, re how not to (necessarily have to) speak in religious tongues.

Dr Robert Buckman is a UK-trained oncologist working in Toronto, Canada. He is well known as a former TV presenter and radio personality, as well as the author of a number of books. In the 1970's he contracted an auto-immune disease and nearly died. 'What my illnesses did was make me braver about talking to patients,' he says. As Associate Professor at the University of Toronto, he teaches communication skills to medical students and doctors, particularly in the area of breaking bad news.

One of the things he focuses on is a strategy to get doctors to address and acknowledge 'the emotion in the room' (the most difficult aspect of communication according to surveys of oncologists and something that most doctors ignore). Several studies show that how a doctor communicates not only has an impact on patients' satisfaction with their overall care, but also on their adherence to recommended treatments and overall health outcomes.

Now that we know that all things that Christ did, he did for all of creation, and not just for the Christians, we are well placed to engage both God's creation and more of God himself. There are many ways by which this divine agreement can happen: a handshake of affirmation following a successful operation; a silent moment, held in response to a patient's challenging diagnosis; or a mother nearing death, asking the question of a practitioner, 'how can I tell my children?'

It is in these kinds of moments that people can sense and feel they are *'known'* by their practitioner (yes, in part); as per Paul words: *'now that you have come to know God, or rather to be known by God'* (Gal. 4:9). In the same way that we seek to follow the wind of the Spirit (as per Jn. 3:8), so too, we can follow the emotion unfolding within a consult, so as to respond and evoke that power of divine agreement. It is in this way that both patient and practitioner can, should they decide, each express more of their story in God. Reading this, it seems to me that subjectivity can be quite a good tonic for those who desire health and healing!

For those who seek to engage the remedial space design of creation, they need to know that the healing room journey is not tracked on the basis of medical interventions or medications. As is often the case with, for example, cancer patients (should that cancer continue over time), the experiences and reflections that arise in the person will become much more prominent in their life than the medical part of their experience. This to say that medical input has an important role to play, but it is not the greater part of what is happening in the creation sphere of healthcare and healing.

three power plays

In our exploration of the remedial space we looked at the progression by which a person engages the experience. Let's again follow this progression; this time via the assistance of Philippians 3:10-11. There Paul says, re Christ, *'that I may know him and the power of his resurrection and the fellowship of his sufferings, being conformed to his death; in order that I may attain to the resurrection from the dead'*. This progression from Philippians – ie suffering, death, resurrection – is one and the same as that which happens in the remedial space experience; should the person in view decide to go in the right direction, ie into life. Before I proceed further into this Philippians progression, I will take an opportunity to align Romans 8 with Philippians 3.

ROMANS MEETS PHILLIPIANS

The first step into the remedial space experience in both texts is *'suffering [in fellowship] with him'* (Rom. 8:17 and Phil. 3:10). The second step has to do with our experience of decay and the ultimate demise of all temporal forms, which leads to *'futility... in hope'* (Rom. 8:20). This aligns with our being *'conformed to his death'* (Phil. 3:10). The third shared step is described in Romans 8:22 as a *'birth'*; in Philippians it is referred to as *'resurrection'*, which, ultimately, has to do with the unseen/fullness being released from creation into humanity. Note: Kenneth Weust (1893-1962), a well known New Testament Greek scholar, refers to the word, *'resurrection'*, in Philippians, as our coming into newness of life in this age, and from there leading into the age to come.

What is in view here, re Philippians 3:10-11, is an opportunity to be aware and responsive to the client's experience of *'suffering'* (with Christ, Rom. 8:17), and *'death'* (ie separation, letting go, eg Jn. 12:24), and *'resurrection'* (into newness of life). Yes, of course, there is the physical aspect of this equation; but here I am referring to the unseen relational part of the person's unfolding story in God. This three-fold progression is happening most all of the time in every place on earth. Among other things, this progression speaks of that forward movement into creation, as per Job's experience into more of God's creation.

In this *'wise'* and *'harmless'* approach, the practitioner does not necessarily have to spend a minute or even a few seconds trying to work out which of the three Philippians' steps the client is currently on; this to say that you don't have to try too hard to fathom it all. Instead, trust in the truth that both you and the client are made in God's image and made from God's creation. From there, you can follow the emotion in the room; you can use your intuition and/or your instincts; you can look at a client's face and gauge their fear and/ or their hopes – in all, you can be commonly human and engaged in the divine.

It is the person you are that makes the difference. Your presence, along with that power of agreement from God in your midst, can change the atmosphere for the good. This can happen, even if we often fail or falter in our attempts at righteousness. It is this encounter that generates a setting by which a person's story in God can be, in part, known and voiced. As I have said, the remedial space experience is intrinsic to one's ongoing story in God. As such, this same encounter, as per above, is able to establish a context within which the remedial space progression can more fully emerge; not just in the person, but also in the space (the heavens) of a consulting room or a hospital. In regards to this wise and harmless approach to the Genesis mandate, I would suggest we keep following Jesus, who said: *'take care how you listen; for whoever has, to him more shall be given'* (Luke 8:18).

FOR THOSE OF A PRACTICAL BENT

I do feel that I have been somewhat remiss when it comes to practical applications of what I have been talking about in this chapter. So, with a view to showing off some of my practical bent, I will, for those who are interested, suggest some questions that might be used in a consult to help draw out the person's story in God (with a particular view to the Philippians' description of the remedial space progression). In what follows, do forgive me, should I engage in over-much hand holding. I am aware that most of these questions will be familiar to healthcare workers. Again to say, it's about the person; not just the words.

Here follows the starters: 'it must be difficult for you to take this burden on at this time in your life'; 'do you think this health issue might possibly bring about changes to your lifestyle, for the good?'; 'were there any lifestyle pressures that you think might have contributed to this illness?'; 'what might be some of the challenges to you and your family that could arise from this diagnosis?'; 'what changes have you experienced in your life because of this condition?' Or, for the brave: 'what are your thoughts and feelings about your condition?' or 'do you have any thoughts about why this illness might have happened?' Enough! Do feel free to add or subtract to this list.

_____

know the room you're in

There was a lot more in this chapter that I wanted to include; but it was too much. So I let it go. At this stage, I still don't know what the archetypal nurse might say in regards to time restraints, re the introduction of the remedial space design and its purpose. My mention of minutes and seconds, in regards to responding to the patient in the room should, possibly, get a positive response from the nurse – maybe!

I would also think that the archetypal doctor would be pleased that religion would not (directly) impact on the medical. Also, I would hope that practitioners, reading this book, will be encouraged to further engage their Christian beliefs in the relational and spiritual dimensions of their work. Dr Cate Hayes, I am sure, would most certainly be an advocate of this kind of approach to healthcare and healing.

And for those who are chaplains or working in counselling or pastoral care, yes, there is scope for them to ask more questions and give more space to conversations that touch on the things we have considered here. This to say that these professions have different sets of rule and authority to that of medicine-based disciplines. Thus the need for those in different disciplines, who believe, to *be fitted and held together by that which every joint supplies* (Eph. 4:16).

white stone readied

Once we know that disease is more than just disease, and pain is more than just pain, and that suffering is not just divine judgement, and death has a purpose beyond just wrath, then what we search out and agree on together on this earth can help us make a whole lot more sense of life and death. This is why a *'word fitly spoken'* (Prov. 25:11 AV) by a practitioner to a patient can make a difference – to *'all things'*.

Your own and other peoples' story is not an epitaph on a dead man's grave; rather it has to do with the closeness of God to each son and each daughter who has and holds their breath in him. Your story speaks of your faith and the fullness you have gathered. Again to say, this is not so much because you have *'come to know God'* (which is a good start), but more so because you have become more *'known by God'* (Gal. 4:9); known in the sufferings, the deaths and the fulsome resurrections these seed into your life eternal.

It was Jesus who said: *'To him who overcomes I will give him a white stone, and a new name written on the stone which no one knows but he who receives it'* (Rev. 2:17). This is the deepest, most intimate, most telling part of your story in him. Thus the need, indeed the call, to engage in good conversations (seen and unseen – heard or silent) in the healing rooms of creation; this with a view to our doing our part, in God, to work all things and all persons together for the good – this, of course, in line with that amazing Genesis mandate.

To unlock more of this vast creation mandate to fill the earth in its every dimension, I now proceed again to Ephesians chapter 3:9-11. These amazing verses weep in the waiting, crying out to us, saying that we must *'bring to light what is the administration of the mystery which for ages has been hidden in God who created all things; [this] so that the manifold wisdom of God might now be made known through the church to the rulers and the authorities in the heavenly places. This... in accordance with the eternal purpose which he [God] carried out in Christ Jesus our Lord'*. This divine strategy is all about your work in healthcare; hence the need for this key creation sphere to activate and release its divine wisdom from earth to sky to heaven's eyes – are we ready?

14

Divine Wisdom
for the Church in Creation

I left us in the prior chapter speaking about what I believe to be the most comprehensive description of God's strategy for humankind; this from Ephesians 3:9-11. It is a most strange description of things and events, designed in such a way that God's *'eternal purpose'* (Eph. 3:11) will be realised. The core of this plan is that we take hold of *'the manifold wisdom of God'* and make it *'known... to the rulers and authorities in the heavenly places'* (Eph.3:10). And what kind of strategy is that? Well, apparently, it's God's strategy; so we best pay attention!

I have peppered this part of Ephesians in a number of paragraphs in this book, so as to acclimatise the reader to this often overlooked strategy for the body of Christ (and, thereby, the strategy for all humanity). To put another peg in the ground of earth, re this passage from Ephesians 3:9-11, I will say a few words about those *'rulers and authorities in the heavenly places'*. This will help us to more clearly set the context for what proceeds in this and the following chapter. The phrase *'heavenly places'*, refers, of course, to Hebraic cosmology, as per, *'in the beginning God created the heavens and the earth'* (Gen. 1:1). In chapter four of this book I made mention of the three heavens – the first, human; the second, angelic; and the third, God's Throne. It would follow from this that God wants us – ie you and I – to make known his *'manifold wisdom'* to the inhabitants of all three heavens.

It's so obvious, but it needs to be said: God's eternal purpose is so amazing, so much so that it can only be God. I mean, how on earth could a person posit such a thing as this? How is it possible for, say, John and Mary and Fred and Stacey to head off into the cosmos with a dollop of wisdom in their luggage to spread around, say, in the middle heaven? It's no wonder so many theologians move somewhat quickly past this text; with many saying that Paul is referring here to Jesus being more powerful than *'Artemis [or Dianna] of the Ephesians'* (Acts 19:34). But this is not about a beauty or a power contest; it is about the Genesis mandate and God's strategy to get it done. In this chapter I will focus on the *'manifold wisdom of God'*, and in the following chapter I will complete our consideration of this Eph. 3:10 strategy.

what's wisdom got to do with it?

So, what is a *'manifold wisdom'*? My first response to that is to distinguish between truth and wisdom. To my mind, wisdom is truth at work in creation. By way of example, there are lots of truths we have considered in the book. But it's only when we close the book and get on with working in line with these truths that we will be eligible to possibly wear the badge of *'manifold wisdom'*. Paul's use of the word, *'manifold'*, suggests that this wisdom has many folds in its divine garment; as in, God's wisdom is not just one thing; rather, it is many-faceted. I dare not try to define what this wisdom is, but I can, in part, describe some of its expressions. It partakes of the good, ie the qualitative good; it pertains to the work; it is relational, not dogmatic; it reveals God's invisible attributes, divine nature and eternal power; and it results in generosity, born of love. Readers, of course, will no doubt add their own thoughts to this list.

Another attribute of a manifold wisdom is that it has been at one time hidden; this so that it might be found. It appears that the one who is hiding all this potential wisdom is God, himself – as per the following statements: *'the mystery which for ages has been hidden in God'* (Eph. 3:9) and *'It is the glory of God to conceal a matter, but the glory of kings [ie us, the "royal priesthood"] is to search out a matter'* (Prov. 25:2) and *'I will utter things hidden since the foundation [of creation]'* (Matt. 13:35 ILGE). Again to say, God does enjoy a good game of hide and seek!

What we see again here is yet another spoil to the idea that God's plan, pre and post-Fall, is mostly about the curse, the wrath and the punishment, and from there, get saved, keep moral and wait for heaven. Again to say, most Christians do not live as if this is true; because it's not; in that this version of reality cannot sustain meaning in life. That is why hardly anyone I know who is a Christian lives that way. But, for them, that's not the end of their suppression; this because they are held in check by the yoke of morality. What do I mean by that?

Morality is essential, but it can only inform us of moral boundaries, should we transgress them. Morality does not, because it cannot, define or engage the qualitative good within those boundaries. In this regard, note Paul's words from Rom. 2:15, concerning the law of God within a person. He speaks of a person's *'conscience bearing witness, and their thoughts alternately <u>accusing</u> or else <u>defending</u> them'*. Note that words like 'affirming' or 'valuing' are not used in this context. I stress this point because, all too often, saints look at the word 'good' (as in, *'good work'*) and think that it means 'moral'. But imagine God, on the sixth day, looking on at all his creation work and saying, it is moral! If we keep focused on morality as our measure of spirituality, it will come at the expense of our creativity, ie our inheritance in creation. In this regard, note the progress of the Ephesians thief, from stealing to contributing – as per Eph. 4:28. So then, where is this manifold wisdom to be found?

cosmology, stills, matter and young

If one wants to play this divine game of hide and seek, they will at first need to have some understanding of the landscape, as per, *'in the beginning...'* (Gen. 1:1). You see, the very design of God's creation is such that it gives us lots of clues to the whereabouts of wisdom. Of course, it won't always be simple to unearth these treasures. There are many challenges along the way – thorns, sweat, relationships, decay, disease, death, to name a few. The good news is, however, that these challenges frequently point the way through to wisdom treasures.

Most innovations (ie possible new wisdom) throughout history have arisen from a person's understanding of the universe, be that by design or default. This, of course, is self-evident – in that a person cannot but respond to what they believe is reality. In chapter one I noted the impact of Aristotle and Copernicus on our modern-day understanding of the universe. Also in this cosmological mix is Plato's dualistic version of the universe, which was taken up eagerly by the early Catholic Church, with all its resultant follow-on effects. I also mention Darwin, who anchored his idea of the 'survival of the fittest' in the natural realm. Yes, he believed that God was ultimately the maker of this idea; but, again, its verification had to do with his beliefs about the natural universe. And then there is Paul the Apostle who, as I have said, validated the Gospel on the basis of creation's design – as per Rom. 1:19-20.

I am aware, of course, that most people do not link their understanding of the universe with their healthcare issues. But if they did, it might come as a surprise to them that their state of health is, in fact, a by-product of the big bang. As in, suffering, decay and death are, in essence, just a part of 'collateral damage' in the universe! This last statement might sound a bit unkind; but that is an issue for those who believe that version of reality. Clearly, it is important that we decide which version of the cosmos we are tuned into. To say it another way: make sure your software fits with both your hardware and its operating system.

I am very pleased to announce that the ancient Hebraic cosmology is the only cosmology I know of in which health and healing are intrinsic, ie purposely built-in. Yes, this statement will sound bizarre to Western secular sensitivities. And that's just fine! But to say, this ancient Hebraic vision of the universe can also generate new thinking, and thus, new wisdom – indeed, *'manifold wisdom'*. This sight of life is more than able to establish a fertile and living context within which good wisdom for healthcare and healing can emerge. Let's look at possible beginnings from such a sight as this.

THE SOUND THEREOF

I (Thwaites) was a speaker at a healthcare conference in the UK (Christian oriented). In my sessions I began to unpack the idea of the remedial space design of creation. It, thankfully, was well received. After my second talk, two doctors came up to me. One of them said that they were very excited at the content of my talks. I asked them what they were particularly excited about. I remember that they both talked together in response to my question. They said that they had been working in Africa over a number of years, treating people who have HIV AIDS. They had both felt that something larger was happening sociologically and spiritually than just this virus. I asked them what it was, and they responded, saying (paraphrased): we don't know; but when we heard your talk about creation as a healing space, we began to feel that this had to do with what we were trying to see or engage. I had to go, but I so wanted to stay and talk with them. But I didn't see them after that. So, if one or other of you gets this book, then do let me know what has happened since!

in search of painful wisdom

I have mentioned the importance of language, along with cosmology; and the need to break down dualism in our minds, so as to bring in a more integrated understanding of life in God's good creation. The above account points us in that same direction. This language is not far from us; indeed, it is as close as the Scriptures itself. With that in view, my plan is to press in to some of the issues we have covered in this book, so that we might learn to apply them to that Ephesians 3:9-11 text; this so as to establish a creation context within which this 'manifold wisdom of God' might be better known and thus engaged. Let's begin with God's wisdom for pain and its close cousin, suffering.

Many medical doctors (and therapists) I have worked with or spoken to at workshops and conferences get quite nervous when it seems to them that I might be making a virtue of pain and suffering. Most certainly, this is challenging territory, both medically and psychologically. More so for those engaged in medical care, the idea that pain might (or should) continue when there is opportunity for pain relief can seem abhorrent to them. As such, I hasten to say that suffering in itself is most certainly not a virtue. My issue here has to do with the meaning of pain and its divine purpose; this with a view to hopefully generating some of that 'manifold wisdom'.

From our exploration thus far in this book, we have learned a number of things from the Scriptures about pain and suffering, as per the following. Pain and weakness, be they from disease, physical demise or injury, serve to ignite, shape and texture our experience of suffering in the inner person. Pain relief, when it comes, forges a bond between practitioner and patient. Eve's multiplied pain in childbirth served as a means by which humanity and creation could continue in step with each other. Pain guides and intensifies the process of human birth. In regards to the remedial space design, pain relief is able to open up a larger space within which the person involved can consider their way of life. Our sufferings in Christ serve to release our God-given inheritance, via the birth pangs they generate within creation. As such, pain guides both creation and humanity through into the birth of the fullness, ie the culmination of this age. Pain is a strange, hard and wonderful companion in this journey of life. In this regard, I note the book, The Gift of Pain, by Dr Paul Brand, who worked for decades with people afflicted by leprosy (Hansen's disease); it is well worth the read.

Again to say, what I am doing here is to draw out particular truths from Scripture, with a view to establishing a creation context for considering different or various approaches to the meaning and purpose of this critical part of God's plan for humans. Again, this exploration is situated off-line to the medical academy,

> *'Enlarge the place of your tent; stretch out the curtains of your dwellings, spare not; lengthen your cords and strengthen your pegs'*
> Isaiah 54:2

so as to enlarge the scope of our enquiry into the larger creation sphere of healthcare and healing.

it's time for bunches to blossom

Imagine a bunch of healthcare workers, off-line, at a two day retreat, exploring the place of pain and suffering in God's plan for humans. In this they would have in their sights the same cosmology that Jesus had when he walked in Palestine all those years ago. Let's say that a person in that bunch, (say) Ruth, was interested in Hebrews 5:14, which reads: *'solid food is for the mature, who because of practice have their senses trained to discern good and evil'*. Ruth asked the group what they thought about this verse. In response, another person, Stephen, said that the writer of Hebrews must have known there is a link between the stimuli received by the senses of the body and the disposition of the inner person.

Helen responded, saying that this means that pain signals in the body are able to turn into suffering in a person's mind and emotions, and that this must be quite important to God's purpose. Yes, said Jack, I read something like this in Romans 8:17; if you don't suffer with Christ, you will not be able to take hold of your inheritance in God. Now I can understand more about what Paul was saying in that verse. Bill was hungry, and said that it was time for lunch. Penny said that we should utilise the afternoon and evening sessions to explore what we might be missing or needing to take hold of, in regards to God's plan for pain and suffering; this (she said), not only for ourselves, but also for the people we engage as patients or clients. Bill said, amen, and the rest nodded hungrily.

in search of accelerated learning

The above mythical bunch seemed to be rather quick off the theological mark, re the issues at hand. The reality is, however, that events like these often move quite slowly; mostly because the participants are still theologically centered in their 'church gathered' culture. Thus my desire to put pen to paper, in the hope of priming the theological pump, in further hope that from little wheels, big wheels might begin to turn within the Christian mind.

WHEELS WITHIN WHEELS

I did an evening event, re this material, and began by saying that there was pain in the pre-Fall Garden of Eden. On hearing this, a woman looked at me in a kind of shock, and said to me that pain could not be in Eden before the Fall because it was a place of peace and safety and God's presence. I then mentioned about Eve's multiplied pain post-Fall; saying that if there was no pain in the pre-Fall Garden, then how could it be multiplied in post-Fall period. She got it straight away and, with a different kind of shock now settling on her face, her Christian universe was overturned in a moment of time. Yes, it's true: little wheels can help make big wheels turn.

I have come alongside a number of healthcare workers, in that off-line setting, engaging them theologically in regards to their work, their desire and their strategies to accomplish that good working desire. In this one to one setting it is easier to progress in language and learning, re the Hebrew vision. One such person is Dr Chris Hayes. Over many years he and I have explored how the remedial space design might change and/or develop his approach to the practice of pain management. I won't go into detail here, but I do believe that his approach to pain constitutes a manifold wisdom. Of course, he would not say that; one reason being that hardly anyone knows what it means! Here follows a snapshot of a shift in his work in pain management, from a more linear to a more wholistic approach to his work.

The Integrated Pain Service I manage has developed a graphical representation that enables patients to consider the meaning of their pain and participate in holistic management. This model seeks to hold a tension between six domains: physical, emotions, thoughts, social, environmental and spiritual. This avoids the Platonic temptation to divide off any one domain and give it pre-eminence.

It is an interesting exercise to work around each domain in turn and consider examples of its 'type' of thinking. 'Pain is all about a ruptured disc'. 'Pain is all about the outworking of anxiety or depression'. 'Pain is all about unhelpful cognitive styles such as catastrophysing'. 'Pain is all about the pursuit of gain in the worker's compensation system'. 'Pain is all about sin or demonic oppression'. The model invites a holding of tension rather than division and an exploration of the complex ways in which pain presents in each domain and how these domains then interact with each other.

Dr Chris Hayes
Pain Management Specialist, Newcastle, Australia

---

wisdom from pathogens

Let's now take a look at God's wisdom for pathogens. Again, we do this so that we might establish a creation context for our theological understanding of disease bearing organisms and viruses. Note: I will use the word 'disease' in this section to refer to pathogenic disease; unless otherwise advised. Again, this is not a comprehensive enquiry into disease, but rather a catalyst or a trigger for an enquiry into life and death, in God. So, here comes the brief.

Medical science has been trying to get rid of disease for a long time now. In the early days, when penicillin first got under way, there was hope that in time they would be overcome and be no more. Alas, more and more, we have had to come to terms with the fact that our pathogenic adversarial allies are much more wily and intelligent than we ever could have imagined. They just won't lie down and die for the human race! There have been some great battles won, but the war on disease seems never-ending.

These diseases are very resistant in the face of our ongoing medical military operations. As such, perhaps it is time we engage this resistance and begin a new round of negotiations. It is only recently that warnings about over-use of antibiotics have been issued by medical authorities. This, however, is not done so much with a view to a new approach to disease and its purpose; rather, it is more the case of better the disease you know than the super-disease you don't – and thus cannot cure.

Be we saint or secular, if we continue to think that diseases are just random acts of a Darwinian universe, or worse, a product of divine wrath, or even worse, a product of the devil, we will believe in line with our choice. If, however, we have an inkling that we are dealing with an adversarial ally, one that takes us on with a purpose that is ultimately for the good, then different choices can emerge, and from that, more wisdom can arise.

Disease is something we are not meant to totally destroy (as if we could!). Rather, we are meant to subdue it, with a view to ruling over it; this so that disease can express and engage its particular creation purpose, which in turn, of course, will serve us in our created purpose. This is not about some kind of medical passivism! We are meant to take pathogens on, rather than just letting them have their opportunistic way in us. Both our immune system and various medications kill millions upon millions of organisms and viruses each day, each hour, each minute; this to say that just like our human bodies, these pathogens also have a use-by date.

There's a whole lot of divine wisdom ready to be downloaded from these key truths of Scripture. Yes, there will come a time when the medical war will find it peace. We just need to ensure it is the right kind of peace! On a personal note, as a lay-person (not a medical practitioner), I live in hope that no one finds a cure for the common cold; this, because its replacement might well kill us all!

the dangers of collapsed distinctions

From the challenge of pain, pathogens and suffering, I turn now to another significant issue (that I have not canvassed in this book). It relates to a growing trend in modern medicine that goes by the name, 'material determinism'. This, to my mind, is one of those *'speculations and... lofty thing[s] raised up against the knowledge of God'* (2 Cor. 10:5). As I have said, Aristotle's legacy has bequeathed to medical science a singular focus on material forms; leaving little or no room for the unseen to be expressed. Again to say, this has its benefits in a pluralistic society.

The discipline of modern science often equates in peoples mind with naturalism, ie all there is is matter and energy – no divine, no spiritual. Truth is, however, that many scientists who explore the material world are not philosophical naturalists. Rather, they are people who believe in more than matter and energy, ie they believe in transcendence or the divine or the spiritual. The pure naturalists, however, are getting a bit too excited by their own advertising, as per the following:

MODERN MEDICINE RIDS HUMANITY OF TRANSCENCENCE

The neurobiologist, Dr Lone Frank, says that *'Understanding patterns of activity in our 100 billion brain cells is set not only to transform our understanding of faith, but also economic decision-making, morality, addiction, love, violence, law enforcement, marketing and happiness'*. Her conclusion is that *'the existence of God does not become more evident with time. To the contrary, the data is overwhelmingly indicating that the sacred is found between the ears'* (quotes from article, Sydney Morning Herald Newspaper, May 15th, 2010).

Lone Frank's account indicates to us where medical science is (or might be) heading. Frank's beliefs highlight the need for those of us who appreciate transcendence to get to know more about what we do believe about disease, decay, death and the nature and purpose of suffering these bring to humanity. This to say, we need to decide on our macro-medical/healthcare model. The determinists it seems are determined to close down much of the relational and subjective facets of medicine. If healthcare loses these, then much of its breath will be lost, and that, most surely, will not be healthy for healthcare!

If Lone Frank was to proceed to remake my brain, I wonder in whose image she would make it? First up, she would need to have a good idea of just what a good-looking brain might look or feel like. The trouble she will have here is that the idea of a 'good-working brain' is something that is subject to her own beliefs; which she says is, in turn, subject to brain function; which, in turn, is subject to the very beliefs that are (apparently) that brain function itself!

I wonder how long it will take the tiger spinning in this circle of fractured logic to turn to butter! It is one thing to map your neurological pathways or, for that matter, sequence your genes – but it's an altogether other thing to capture and extinguish the 'inner person' in the process. The first and forlorn casualty of this silo of circular logic is that the subjective and the objective are collapsed into a monism. Knowing that your beliefs are 'of faith' is that which enables you to keep moving between fact and faith, seen and unseen, object and subject, physical and spiritual, plus more. We must not collapse these living distinctions. As such, long live the divine 'one with/distinct from' paradox!

exponential wisdom

Whether at this stage in the book we are encouraged, angry, indifferent, confused, tired or mixed, we are all left with the same questions. What is the meaning of pain and suffering? Why does disease have to exist? Why do humans have to die? How can a child be born deformed? And so on it goes. Thankfully, none of us have all the answers, excepting God. That is why I hold on to the verse from Exodus 4:11, which says: *'who has made man's mouth? Or who makes him dumb or deaf, or seeing or blind? Is it not I, the Lord?'* This might well sound trite in the face of misery and death, but where else can you go – not to the devil, not to the curse, not to Darwin's fittest, and not to predestination – but, rather, to God, who made all things, for a purpose.

Often the life of the person who is facing their own death is taken away by over-much medical intervention. It's like they are forcing life to keep on happening and not allowing death to occur. When this happens the life that the person wants to express in that part of their story can be taken away from them. If we could rediscover our intuition of what was really happening, we could do more of the hand holding and support and keep the space open for life conversations. That would be a blessed thing in many ways.

Dr Chris Hayes
Pain Management Specialist, Newcastle, Australia

God is judge, God is life – and in the same time that I said those two phrases, hundreds of millions of flowers have died. I say this to say that it seems that God is not as invested in the long-term 'seen' physical dimension, as much as many would like him to be. It appears, however, that he places a lot more emphasis on the unseen, which, as we know, aligns fully with his eternal nature. To my mind, this is one of the most acute and telling truths we need to embrace.

It is a hard truth; but one that holds the words we need to unlock a whole lot more *'manifold wisdom'* for human disease, suffering and death. There is, of course, lots more wisdom than this on offer; indeed all three heavens over that one earth exists to bring this wisdom, along with us, to more of life. So then, let's keep moving through these heavens, so as to *'press on toward the goal for the prize of the upward call of God in Christ Jesus'* (Phil. 3:14). Let's keep growing up into him.

15

Healthcare Rulers and Authorities
in Heavenly Places

We have looked through various lenses in this book, so as to better understand God's person and purpose. The largest finite context for our enquiry into healthcare and healing has been God's creation, in both its physical and spiritual dimensions. To bring us very close to the end of this book I will look through two more lenses, they being the church and the angels. I again will seek to meld these two big players in God's plan to the Ephesians 3:9-11 text we have been considering; this, so as to complete our enquiry (in this book at least) into the divine strategy for humans in creation.

First the church, then to angels. In the Ephesians 3:9-11 text we read that it is *'the church'* that will *'make known... the manifold wisdom of God... to the rulers and the authorities in the heavenly places'*. So then, what is the church and, also, where it is located? In chapter two of this book I briefly mentioned that God designed the church to be a body of people standing in Christ in every sphere of life in creation. I want to now expand on that cosmological primer.

the whereabouts of church

To begin, I will mention a friend of mine who once said: 'whoever gets the name church, wins'. It's a wicked statement, with quite some sting in its tail; it being a political statement, in that it pertains to the nature of authority and rule over our present forms of church, particularly institutional forms. It was Jesus who said, *'I will build my church, and the gates of hell shall not prevail against it'* (Matt. 16:18 AV). I wonder what kind of church Jesus was thinking about when he said this to his disciples. To find out, let's start with the church as we presently know it. A typical church is concentrated on gatherings of Christians in a building or a home, led by a minister of religion who directs activities such as preaching, outreaches, pastoral care and fund-raising. All good things. Implicit in this form of church is that it is seen to exist at the core of God's plan for humans. Its general strategy is to fan-out from this church core in the hope of gaining more impact for Christ in the broader community. It is a well tried and straightforward template with a very long history. So then, what might happen if we applied some cosmological scrutiny to this form of church, in regards to its location and divine mission?

In my reading of Scripture, there are three main descriptions of the church – in regards to what it is and where it is (as distinct from what might or might not do). I have mentioned the first description, were Jesus said, '*I will build my church...* [and so on]' (Matt. 16:18). The second description is from 1 Timothy 3:15, where Paul speaks of the '*household of God, which is the church of the living God, the pillar and support of the truth*'. The third is found in Ephesians 1:22-23, where we read that God the Father '*put all things in subjection under [Christ's] feet, and gave him as head over all things to the church, which is his body, the fullness of him who fills all in all*'. Let's now push further into our cosmological analysis.

In the first description, Jesus is seen pitching the church at the '*gates of hell*', confident that it will prevail against these devilish gates. One wonders, where are these gates situated? Paul knew; he said in Eph. 6:12 that '*our struggle is... against the rulers, against the powers, against the world forces of this darkness, against the spiritual forces of wickedness <u>in the heavenly places</u>*'. So then, the church that Jesus is building is located in the heavenly places – that's interesting.

The next description, that being '*the household of God, which is the church of the living God...*[and so on]' (1 Tim. 3:15), seems to be firmly grounded on the earth, situating itself in a family-like '*household*' setting. This aligns closely with our present-day pattern of church, focused on households or congregational settings. As I said, this form of gathered church sees itself as situated at the core of God's plan for humankind.

What is of particular interest to me, in regards to this 1 Timothy verse, is the phrase '*the pillar and support of the truth*' – as in, the church itself is a pillar and support of truth. I will put aside the mention of '*the truth*' for now, so as to focus on this interesting description of church. To put it plainly, how can the church be at the core of God's plan and at the same time be its *'pillar and support'*? By definition, a pillar and support in a building cannot also be the entire building itself – as in, you cannot have it both ways. I will come back to this possible puzzle soon.

location, location, divine location

It is now Ephesians' turn to tell us about the church. In passing, to say that this epistle is often named as 'the book of the church'. As a lead in to Ephesians 1:22-23, I will refer to vs 20, where Paul says that God *'raised [Christ] from the dead, and seated him at his right hand in the heavenly places'*. There's that phrase again – heavenly places. It must be a very popular location indeed! Another thing to say, before we land on vs 22 of Eph. 1, has to do with the Hebrew prophet, Isaiah, who firmly believed that *'heaven is [God's] throne and the earth is [God's] footstool'* (Isa. 66:1). Again the issue of location pops up.

It would stand to reason that where God the Father is, God the Son would not be too far away. So it is that we read that God the Father *'put all things in subjection under [Christ's] feet, and gave him as head over all things'* (Eph. 1:22); this to say that Christ now stands, with this Father, from the footstool of earth all the way to God's Throne. It would also stand to reason that where Christ is, his church should never be far away. Hence Paul's next words, which speak of God as giving his Son *'to the church, which is his [ie Christ's] body'* (ibid vss 22-23). To further follow suit, it would stands to reason that where humanity in Christ is, then the Genesis mandate to *'fill the earth'* will (or should) be ever-present. Hence Paul's final words in this chapter, that Christ's *'body [you and I are] the fullness of him who fills all things in all things'* (vs 23 ILGE). Now that's what you call a big church!

To say it again: the church that Jesus came to build exists right now between the ground of earth through the heavenly places, all the way up to touch the Throne of God in the third heaven – all in Christ, who is in God. It is this church, standing in creation, in Christ, that is made to *'bring to light what is the administration [ie the stewardship] of the mystery which for ages has been hidden in God, who created all things'* (Eph. 3:9). Here follows a graphic of what we have considered here. The reader will also note the inclusion of the words 'marriage', 'family' and 'work' in this illustration. I will explain that part of the graphic further on in this chapter. It's time now to see the church.

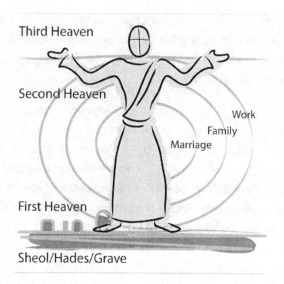

CALVIN COMES CLOSE, BUT NOT CLOSE ENOUGH

The Reformer, John Calvin (1509-1564AD), came close to seeing this church in creation. He described the church Paul referred to in Ephesian 1:22-23 as the universal church of the living and the dead. The challenge for Calvin, I believe, is that he tried to make sense of this passage of Scripture via a Platonic template. And so, with the heaven of God dispatched to the afterlife, and with a wispy spirit realm with no known creation co-ordinates attached as its replacement, Calvin narrowed his 'church search' down to earth. There he focused on the tangible form of church as a congregation under leadership; with the preacher at its core and the divine word spoken on Sunday, driving God's plan for planet earth.

---

the pillar that must support

It is more than evident from the Ephesians text that an expression of church, in which Christians locate themselves in a room or a building a few hours or so each week, is a lessor part of God's plan, and not the core part. This is why the church as a *'household of God'* is the *'pillar and support'*, as distinct from it being the church as *'the fullness of him who fills all things in all things'* (vs 23 ILGE). I have not yet commented on the word *'truth'* in the phrase from 1 Tim. 2:15, *'the pillar and support of truth'*. Simply to say, the *'truth'* is Jesus, as per Jn. 14:6. And where then is Jesus? Well, as we know, he is with his Father, present from the footstool of earth to the Throne of God's third heaven.

Sadly, most Christians don't know there is a church standing in creation; and, as such, their measure of church is most all about what happens in congregations and their church-based initiatives. My conviction is that the church gathered as pillar and support will not know the measure of itself until it holds hands with the church as fullness. We need them both to get the eternal purpose to come to pass. There is but *'one body and one Spirit'* (Eph. 4:4). It appears, however, that within that one-ness of church there is found a distinction. To me, this sounds like something the Trinity would organise!

I don't want to give the impression that after two or so thousand years no one has signed up for this church in creation. The reality is that day by day, multiplied millions of believers have families, go to work, relate to friends and, thereby, touch the ground of their inheritance in God. Along with this are billions of people who seek for the good – as per Rom. 2:7. My intent here is to outline and underline the contours and strategies of this vast divine church design. Let's now draw out a little bite of truth from this new distinguished relationship between church as pillar and support and church as fullness – distinct but one; all in hope of more wisdom to come.

the trinity of work

In the Trinity of Father, Son and Holy Spirit, I would say that the church gathered as *'the household of God'* (1 Tim. 3:15) has as its divine expression, *'the Father, from whom every family in heaven and on earth derives its name'* (Eph. 3:14-15). From there, it is Christ's body (ie us), standing in creation that is called out *'to grow up in all things into him who is the head, Christ'* (Eph. 4:15). It is this body, in creation, that needs to be *'fitted and held together by that which every joint supplies'*, so as to bring about *'the proper working of each individual part'*, which in turn will enable *'the growth of the body for the building up of itself in love'* (Eph. 4:16). As we know, the Holy Spirit proceeds from both the Father and the Son; hence the Spirit's task to intercede for the saints as comforter and support in this work – as per Acts 1:8. If we could stick with that Trinitarian strategy, we would surely do well.

Whilst moving along this Trinitarian street, I will speak about the placement of the words, 'marriage', 'family' and 'work', from the above graphic of Christ standing in creation. First up, note the link between Christ and marriage (Eph. 5:22-33); then the link between the Father and the family (Eph. 6:1-4 and Eph. 3:14-15); and then between the sphere of work and the Holy Spirit (Eph.

6:5 and Acts 1:8), who, as we know, empowers that work, ie *'the work of faith with power'* (2 Thess. 1:11). These three spheres, linked respectively to the Trinity, have to do with the mental or psychological structures within human beings and their relationships to others, to creation and to God.

By way of example, God the Father gives us our identity, God the Son gives us our purpose, and the Spirit brings these effects or relations together in the work, as per *'bearing fruit in every good work'* (Col. 1:10). In this process there is also a movement from infanthood to adulthood to death, ie find your identity, engage your purpose, consolidate your work, and, from there, when you die, leave your inheritance to your children – and on the cycle goes and grows. In this, of course, the father or mother that die carry with them their unseen inheritance in God (should it be good). A lot could be said at this point, as to what modern sensitivities might make of this apparently conventional approach, but this is not the time for that.

In summary, you, with others, are the church, against which the gates of hell will not prevail. Yes, I know this brings with it more responsibility for everyday saints, accustomed, as they often are to relying on church leaders to do most of the divine business, along with, of course, mapping the way to heaven. But, apparently, it is God's plan for you and well... everyone else! So we best get with it. Our next step is to welcome the angels into this divine strategic mix. Well, actually, truth be told, they have been here all along; it is we, the church, that have been, shall I say, missing in action. Having now located the whereabouts of Christ and his body, the church, we are ready to meld this angelic sight in with the Eph. 3:9-11 text. In the prior chapter we focused on *'the manifold wisdom of God'*. It's now time to connect that wisdom to the *'rulers and authorities in the heavenly places'*, so as to get *'the eternal purpose'* done.

contacting your angels

We know about humans, and we are known by God; but the angels; who are they when it comes to the divine plan? Let's seek them out. To do this, I need to first clear some of the angelic air. This has to do with an influential sect that was very popular in the early centuries of the Christian era. It was called 'Gnosticism'. Its followers thought that the earth and its inhabitants were made and ruled by an evil demiurge – an angel-like creature. They believed that their pure/divine spirit had been imprisoned in a body of flesh. And to escape this fleshly sentence, they had to get hold of 'special knowledge', which would bring about an initiation, or revelation, that over time (and after death) would free the spirit from the body and the earth and release it back into the pure spirit realm.

One can see the parallels here between Plato and the Gnostics. As such, it is easy to see why the early church, holding close to Plato, integrated many elements of this way of thinking. In this regard, I note that the 2nd century bishop of Rome, Marcion, became a Gnostic and planted many Gnostic churches across the Roman Empire; in the process, blending Christ into their beliefs. Down to this day, I would say that there are still many Gnostic threads woven into the Christian mind.

A prime example of this is the belief that Satan, post-Fall, took control of the earth, along with (apparently) getting hold of the keys of hell and death. The validation of this belief comes from verses such as 1 Jn. 5:19, which says that *'the whole world lies in the power of the evil one'*. The Scriptures, however, make a very clear distinction between the words *'creation'* and *'world'*. We read in Eph. 1:22-23, that Christ's feet are situated, right now, on the ground of earth and, from there, through *'all creation under [God's] heaven'* (Col. 1:23). This is not the devil's domain; rather, this is God's Throne and his footstool. The apostle John says that *'all that is in the world, the lust of the flesh and the lust of the eyes and the boastful pride of life is not from the Father, but is from the world'* (1 Jn. 2:16). This is where the devil has influence; but also, this is where the good angels contest him, on a two to one basis!

DEVILS CAN'T KILL, GOD AND HUMANS CAN

Reading the above, some might be thinking of the phrase in Heb. 2:14, re *'him who had the power of death, that is, the devil'*. Two things in regards to this statement: Firstly, it was the coming of Christ that ensured that at the end of the age the devil would no longer have power in regard to human death. This aligns with Heb. 2:8, as per Christ's coming to ultimately subject all things to himself, but with the qualification that *'now we do not yet see all things subjected to him'*, as in, right now the devil is still roaming the planet and doing this thing; but one fine day, he won't.

Secondly, the devil and his demons cannot directly kill anyone. They can, however, tempt and deceive people into killing others (and themselves). This is evident in the book of Job, where God decided on the matter of death, and not Satan. Fact is that Mary Smith, who is, say, one-hundred and two, has the power to kill people, and that without God's permission. It's no wonder the devil is jealous of humans.

I would hope that this brief overview of the devil has made some readers a little less Gnostic and a lot more Hebraic in their inclinations! Oh, and by the way, Christ has always held *'the keys of hell and of death'* (Rev. 1:18 AV), and still has them down to this day. Let's now rid our minds of the quasi-demiurge and get back to the actual angels of God.

angels within and beyond the body

When *'the heavens and the earth were completed, and all their hosts'* (Gen. 2:1) a crucial relationship was formed between the hosts of heavens and the human inhabitants of the earth. It is evident in Scripture that the heavens are considered to be 'the measure' of what needs to take place on the earth. Jesus speaks of God's will as being done *'on earth, as it is in heaven'* (Matt. 6:10).

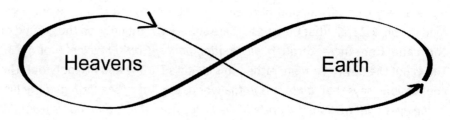

Matthew 18:10 is a very good case in point. It describes a situation in which children on earth are attended by angels, which are said to be *'continually'* beholding the face of God the Father in the heavens. What we see here is a creation reality in which humans, angels and God the Father occupy a shared unseen space together, and that, continually. Again, I mention Paul, who was uncertain as to whether his visit to the third heaven took place *'in the body... or out of the body'* (2 Cor. 12:2). It seems that either of these was an option for the apostle. I referred to this human experience within and through space and time in chapter four and chapter ten of this book.

angels, spheres, territories

What stands out in the angels' job description is their role in upholding the systems or orders that God had established in creation for humanity. These include creation spheres such as marriage, government and family. By way of example, Stephen speaks of the Law, saying to those about to kill him that *'you who received the Law as ordained by angels, and yet did not keep it'* (Acts 7:53). The sense of the word *'ordained'* (Gk. *diatagma*) has to do with establishing and upholding proper order. The word *diatagma* can also be translated as *'decree'* or *'edict'*. Just as court officials or judges or police officers uphold and act in relation to the Law of the land, so too do angels in relation to humanity. I have mentioned the incredible power and purpose of the Law – both in its seen/physical and unseen/relational forms. Just to think, all of the power of this Law is managed and held within the realm of angels, and beyond. It's no wonder they are busy and cannot always stop to talk to us!

Another example: the women of Corinth who cast off their head-coverings, which were a cultural sign (at that time) of their marriage vow (just as, say, the marriage ring is in our time), were informed by Paul that they *'ought to have a symbol of authority on [their] head, because of the angels'* (Cor. 11:10). Note the word *'authority'* here in its relationship to angels. Not only do angels attend to the spheres of creation, eg marriage, they also have a keen interest in what is going on in the territories of the earth, upon which those spheres (and their atmospheres) have their being. This relationship between angels and 'territories' or 'jurisdictions' is found in a number of places in Scripture.

For example, Daniel prayed to God in regards to the future of Israel and an angel was dispatched from the third heaven to convey God's answer. On his way through the middle heaven this angel was met by a strong head wind from one of the fallen 'heavenly-heavies' positioned there. When the angel finally arrived at Daniel's place, he spoke of his journey, saying that *'the prince of the kingdom of Persia was withstanding me for twenty-one days; then behold, Michael, one of the chief princes, came to help me, for I had been left there with the kings of Persia'* (Dan. 10:12-13). Note, in this regard, the correlation between the *'[angelic] prince of the kingdom of Persia'* and *'the [human] kings of Persia'* – re the Eph. 3:10 strategy.

Angels are *'ministering spirits, sent out to render service for the sake of those who will inherit salvation'* (Heb. 1:14). This, among other things, indicates that angels exist for the sake of humanity. This is why angels tend to want to do their job in relation to us, ie they want to share that mutual relational space God designed for *'men [women] and angels'* (1 Cor. 4:9). To make sense of this 'angelic service' we need to keep in mind the above description (from Daniel) of angels as guardians, which have varying degrees of rule and authority over spheres and territories. Let's now take a look at the relationship between Adam and Eve and the good angels.

hand over the rule, powers

When the first couple were made, they were innocent, as in immature, relative to what they might ultimately become. As such, their start point was a long way away from ruling over the birds of the heaven, let alone excelling over the angels of the next heaven. If Adam and Eve had got beyond their apprenticeship in the Garden and headed out into the untamed creation, the angels would have responded to them (ie Adam and Eve) in line with the measure of their standing and maturity in creation. This process was designed so that angels could progressively hand over their God-given power and authority to humans, in line with the particular person's growth and maturity in creation.

I mentioned Psalm 8 several times during this book, re the Genesis mandate. In this text, both humans in general, and *'the son of man'* (Ps. 8:4), Christ, are said to have been *'made... a little lower than the angels'*, with a view to, in time, having *'dominion over the works of [God's] hands'* (Ps. 8:6). It was Christ, who, having *'made purification of sins... sat down at the right hand of the Majesty on high, having become as much better than the angels, as he has inherited a more excellent name than they'* (Heb. 1:3-4).

To put it plainly, angels are made higher in relation to God's Throne than humans are. What is evident from the above texts, however, is that God intends that one day humanity will come to rule over the angelic realm. Remember that Christ came as God the Son made man – fully God and fully human. It was he who came *'as a forerunner for us'* (Heb. 6:20). He took the first human journey from life to suffering to death to resurrection to ascension at the right hand of his Father; and thereby ascended through all of the heavens, including that of the angelic heaven.

As I have said, Christ has done his part, and is now sat down with his Father in the heavenly places. Now it's our turn to stand up and get to work; as in, we are yet to inherit a name that is better than the angels. I note again, the word, *'might'*, in the Eph. 4:10 verse, re Christ *'who ascended far above all the heavens, so that he might fill all things'*. This progressive hand-over of rule and authority from angels to humans holds the key to the Ephesians 3:9-11 divine strategy.

ANGELIC CHAUFEURS

By way of further illustration, re this human/angelic dynamic: a young child does not drive a car, but they are driven places by those who are responsible and competent. When, however, that child grows up they can get their licence, borrow or purchase a car and drive when they want to. So too, angels are designed to hold open and drive these systems of rule and authority; but only as long as it takes for the children of God to attain to a level of maturity that gives them the ability and thus the permission to occupy and drive the vehicle/sphere themselves. When this happens the angels of God are able to hand over the key; and off the young adults go to rule over their own set of wheels and patch of highway. Of course, evil angels will not partake in this divine process.

---

slithers of a serpent not writ large

I used to wonder why that slithering serpent that squirmed its way out of the Garden disappeared for centuries or, possibly, millennia, and then one day surfaced in Job's compound around the times of the Judges. What was *'the prince of the power of the air'* (Eph. 2:2) doing all that time – manufacturing pathogens, designing death, organising his dark minions and their weapons of spiritual destruction?

As I said, angels are made for humans. In this regard, note again Daniel the prophet's experience of the connection between the *'[angelic] prince of the kingdom of Persia'* and *'the [human] kings of Persia'*, as per Dan. 10: 13. You see, without the power of creation and its works there can be no release of angelic rule and authority; this because it is these works that draw out this angelic power. Dark angels cannot do what they want; they can only do what God has made them to do. This is why Satan had to ask permission from God to go after Job. As per the following design:

Creation > kingdom system > good work> back up and hand-over of rule and authority from good angels to the person/s involved.

Creation> world system > evil work> back up and hand-over of rule and authority from evil angels to the person/s involved.

Also to say, the angels of darkness also give us a read out as to where we stand our place of work, or our city, or nation. In this regard I note Paul's approach to Eph. 6, re our struggles *'against the authorities, against the world rulers of this darkness, and against the spiritual hosts of evil in the heavenlies* (vs 12 ILGE). In response to these forces, Paul did not direct the saints to throw volleys of Bible verses at them; nor did he pick up the sword (ie the word of God) and try to take the head off one of those dark heavenly hosts.

Rather, it seems (from Eph. 6:13 on) that Paul wanted the Ephesians to learn how to discern the good/lights and the bad/darkness; this to learn how to assess the measure of those dark powers, so that they, via negation, might come to know more about humanity's general standing in creation – be that in a home, a hospital, a church community, a city or a nation. This aligns with Paul's approach to the dark angelic side. He says in Eph. 5:11-13 that we should *'not participate in the unfruitful deeds of darkness, but instead even expose them; for it is disgraceful even to speak of the things which are done by them in secret. But all things become visible when they are exposed by the light, for everything that becomes visible is light'.*

It's time to leave this angelic interlude; I would hope, however, that we might sing and work with them a lot more often than we presently do. Also, to say, if a good angel is in the room, the atmosphere within that room will feel clear and strong; no scent, but touches of oxygenated wind; ever ready, should needs be, to break into fire.

You are the church; you stand in Christ, from earth through the heavens; you were made to work in line with the Genesis mandate; your work is designed to release wisdom and light into each of the three heavens, so as to release creation's unseen bounty; yes, via ruling humans, angelic authorities and four beasts, and a crystal sea and twenty-four extremely authoritative elders – all situated around God's Throne. It's time, is it not, that we played a whole lot more games of divine hide and seek. Here comes the book-end.

16

May Your Soul Prosper
and Your Body Wear Well

Last chapters can be difficult, particularly for the writer – so little time, and so much more to say! But enough is enough. What follows from here is a quick run through the things, forces, designs and strategies we have considered in this book – this, in hope of a touch of inspiration to take us out, so as to *provoke unto love and to good works'* (Heb. 10:24).

In the first draft version of this book (there have been several) I wrote some encouraging words as a sign off at the end. A few years on I added a few more paragraphs and, yes, even a poem. Further down the track, however, I decided to drop this last chapter, it becoming, in my mind, somewhat unruly.

One of my editors at that time was a doctor of medicine; and in an email, I told her I had decided to get rid of this last chapter. She shot back, saying, 'no way – you have to keep that chapter in'. I had to take her advice; after all, she was the kind of person for which this book was written. So I tidied it up a bit and, since then, I have tried my best to make it presentable. Of course, the reader, for the last time, can judge my efforts. So, enough of the intro, let's get moving.

encouragable!

The body of Christ does not grow up in institutions; rather, it grows up in creation. Like a small seed growing into an immense tree, it moves like leaven through the lump; it works as light in a dark place; its treasure is hidden deep in the earth as well as in, through and over all things. As such, this body does not fear being *'scattered abroad over the face of the whole earth'* (Gen. 11:4). Such a body as this knows its created purpose. As a result, it can move in and grow through every power and authority, with a view to blessing every tribe and nation on earth.

In a time when the weight of unprocessed futility in our systems is such that many are failing and falling, it is important that we be careful. There are many well-intentioned people who are placed in the cracks of the dam and, to mix the metaphor, are told to hold back the night. Certain things need to fall to the ground before new things can emerge. When this happens on a large scale, it is hard, very hard, to know if you should stand and stay or simply leave. In this, give yourself the freedom to choose. Don't try and fix it all; employ emergency measures as needs be. Decide on non-negotiables and seek to clear out or disregard the rest. Maximise your time by making the most of the greater quantity of futility calling your name, with a view to engaging in Christ's sufferings, death and resurrection. It is this journey that will continue to help you know what is real and what is a mirage and what you desire and what you don't.

In the midst of these remedial space experiences, keep on the lookout for new-born resurrection initiatives. When you find them, give what time and resources you can to them. Let your focus stay on your everyday experiences with people and work. It is here you will gain your greatest reward. If a system fails, it does not mean that you have failed. As I said, lots of systems come and go. It is only your works that will remain. Enjoy these works as they present to you each day, in every one of them is your eternal inheritance.

don't fall over your feet

To keep our feet on the earth, whilst we grow though the heavens, we need to look out for the many stumbling blocks that Jesus said will come. To help us here, we will keep idealism out of our house, and thus not become prone to every new round of faddism. We also need to be wary of any and all ideologies; this by refusing to be ruled by any one idea or system of ideas. If you are in a leadership position in your organisation, do not focus on ideology or the idol that often frames it. Instead, keep looking into the unseen attributes, nature and power of your work; remembering that it is the unseen that tells us most about the seen things that physically frame the work we do – not the other way around.

When incompetence or dysfunction arises, consider the role being played by 'futility... in hope'. In these instances, the possibility arises for more 'fractal' occurrences of the remedial space pattern to emerge from your work. As I have said, it is this everyday work that constitutes the largest entry point into the remedial space experience. So, instead of shutting down the remedial space experience by eradicating the problem person or submerging the issue until it explodes at a later date, consider the creational options available to you. It is possible to allow many issues, within reason and depending on the strength or season of the workplace, to play their way out, thereby serving to strengthen the immune system of the body of people engaged in that particular work.

deal well with law

To be free on this 'land' of healthcare, you will need to know that you will never be able to attain to the demands of the moral law of God written in your heart. In this world and in your work you will compromise and you will be compromised; you will love and hate; you will take that which does not belong to you; you will boast and sometimes lie; you will make decisions that bring sadness and harm to people. Sometimes you will do these things because you think you will, in the long run, create a greater good. Other times you will do them because you think your status, your assets or perhaps even your life will be taken away from you if you don't compromise.

Certain church streams continue to assert that it is only when we Christians get holy enough that we will get revival. It's no wonder we are still waiting! Those who really know the Law know that they cannot attain to it. This is why you need to continue to locate your own *'desire for goodness'* (2 Thess. 1:11), and pursue those desires; yes, in the midst of ongoing ethical challenges. In life, we will sometimes be heroic and pay a heavy price for our good exploits. But most of the time it will be just us; speckled and motley with our good and not-so-good intents, along with many shades of the in-between. We may look to certain leaders under lights that appear shiny, ideal and faith-filled, and we may be tempted to believe their advertising. But if we are mature, we will know that they are just like us, part-time heroes, full-time people and all-time saints. In Christ, we are no longer good or bad; we are simply forgiven, adopted and sent into creation.

guard your valuables

It is hard to keep in mind that money is not the measure of one's life; particularly with most everything geared toward it. If, however, a person seeks to serve God rather than mammon, they will experience far greater clarity lighting up their way ahead. If you serve God's creation purposes you will be able to distinguish between money, which is useful, and creation capacity, ie *'the fullness'*, which is essential. If you have enough money you have power to make many earthly things happen instantly. If, however, you have creation capacity, you will be able to work on a much larger scale. Indeed, your work force will include righteous angels and the creation itself.

To keep us moving in the right direction, we will keep in our hearts the truth that all things and thus all people are designed by God to work together for the good. Knowing this, we will be better able to search out the good in all of its attendant joys and suffering; hidden, as they often are, in all kinds of places, be that in a group of people working in medical research; in a nursing unit surviving against all odds; in the heart of a person working within a governing authority; in the smile of a child coming for help and healing; or in the death of person who told his truth and died embracing life. It is as you activate that heart desire for the good that a well-spring of power will cascade through your work with and for others.

Our movement toward the fullness will not mean that any structure will remain or be safe. Through to the end of this age certain systems of humanity will get better and others will get worse, and they will both do so at a faster and faster pace. As we progress through the many and varied containers of this life – different jobs, companies, settings, set-backs, promotions, contracts and contacts – we will be able to move between the forms and keep hold of our growing creation content. Those who are well-practiced in suffering, death and resurrection will be far better placed to travel from one life-phase to the next.

And what then will become of those *'rulers and the authorities in the heavenly places'*? As we make known *'the manifold wisdom of God'* through our life and work, our overtures will be met by a progressive unfolding of creation's fullness. In line with this divine design, as we rise, creation will rise with us. And as it is with creation, so it is with angels. Whilst the wicked angels respond to power structures, the righteous angels respond to good works. The light of these good angels will join with the light we shine through our work, so as to progressively expel the dark angels (not all) from the atmospheres over our homes, our places of work, our schools, church gatherings our cities and more.

As the momentum of our good works proceeds, both creation and angels will join with us in procession toward God heaven. It is here that the present age begins to give way to the age to come. Our life is short, but eternal. We need to work the works of him who sent us in this day and this generation.

There will come a time when the Father declares that it is time for the Son to come again from heaven and crown our works with fullness. At that time there *'comes the end, when he delivers up the kingdom to the God and Father, when he has abolished all rule and all authority and power'* (1 Cor. 15:24). After that happens, what will stand out is that which already stands out from the heavenly perspective – you and the story of your life; you and the unseen attributes, nature and power you have gleaned and gained from all things in the heavens and on the earth.

It is these goods that will be poured into our *'imperishable body'* (1 Cor. 15:42), fitted for the age to come (not to mention the many ages that are still to come – as per Eph. 2:7). Now wouldn't you want to go on a journey like that? Well, truth is, that you and I and all others who breathe are already on this journey. As such, don't forget your torch, your companions, your food, your tent and your map – plus sundry items.

Not to put too much pressure on healthcare workers (we know you are very busy!), but with you being so often close to the cries generated by the hope held within decaying physical forms, we need you to help us unearth a big measure of that *'manifold wisdom'* that God has hidden in the creation sphere of healthcare and healing. This wisdom, born so close to the bone and blood of humans, needs to be poured into other spheres of work. I look forward to the day that business and government and other spheres find lots more healing in themselves, and carry that healing to those they serve. To accomplish this, we need to have lots more of those wisdom finders, ie those bunches that blossom, to arise and take their place in God's given landscape.

many thanks, on earth and in the heavens

Again to comprehend the reality that this creation has been designed by God as one vast healing room of life – one huge remedial space within and from which we can grow and mature in life and in God. This creation design is beyond amazing, but well within our reach. So as to not lose our way, but, rather, fix our cosmological co-ordinates, we need to keep tracking those three cries of Romans 8 – those of the children, the creation and the Spirit (who ever seeks to join the two); all this, so that the children and the creation can be finally released from their bondage to physical decay, into the glory of the eternal God.

I am more than pleased to be able to tell my children (and my friends, sainted or otherwise) that this earth has not been written off, cursed by God and turned into a prison house of divine punishment. Rather, I tell them that God has made creation as our counterpart, thereby giving us an ongoing divine reality check; lest we might lose our way on the way to God's heaven.

Finally, thanks to you healthcare workers (and others in healing professions) for the good work and travail you have accomplished. May you continue to help and heal people through their multiple sufferings, their many deaths and frequent resurrections (and yes, holidays), throughout all of the seasons of life, until breath departs.

May your wisdom continue to light up the atmosphere within and over the creation sphere of healthcare and healing. And may your light help diminish the darkness and bring many to the light of eternal life. Remember, you are made for this!

Oops, I almost forgot the poem!

how long have I been breathing this sleep of death?
One minute, one year, I do not know,
both seem the same on waking.
I could stay enclosed here, but instead I am stirred, awakened,
carried up and onto that same terrain where I once stood
in my control and my fear,
in that same place I lost my power
and fell to ground,
suffering and dissolving my way
into the elements of dust and death
But now with body back, my eyes look to see creation looking at me.
I am fragile, scared of what it might bring my way.
But when I reach for my terror, it is no longer there.
In its place is desire, good strong desire,
one that I thought had died
but now... alive,
this desire lifts me up
to meet the good earth before me.
And as I do, my travail begins,
but it is clear, pure and knows how to give birth.
God's own creation, wise womb of eternal life,
knows this well and welcomes my birth pain
It is more than pleased to release the measure of its fullness
to clothe and adorn that child of good desire,
that measure of labour and work,
with extra rendered for play.
I would not choose to take this journey again
but now I know it chooses me,
so, in this, I do not choose,
I breathe.

Bibliography

Long, W. Meredith, *Health, Healing and God's Kingdom*.
(Regnum Books International, Paternoster Publishing, Carlisle, UK, 2000).

Thielicke, Helmut, *Theological Ethics*
(William B. Eerdmans Publishing, Grand Rapids, Michigan, USA, 1964, Second Ed. 1979).

Erickson, Millard J, *Christian Theology*
(Baker Book House, Grand Rapids, Michigan, USA, 5th Printing 1998).

Berkouwer, G. C., *Studies in Dogmatics, Sin*
(William B. Eerdmans Publishing, Grand Rapids, Michigan, USA, 1971, reprint 1980).

Canfield, C. E. B., *The International Critical Commentary on the Holy Scripture of the Old and New Testaments. The Epistle to the Romans, Volume 1,*
(T. & T. Clark, Edinburgh, UK, 1975, reprint 1985).

Bavinck, Herman, *The Doctrine of God*
(The Banner of Truth Trust, Carlisle, Pennsylvania, USA, 1977, reprint 1979).

Brown, Colin, editor, *New International Dictionary of New Testament Theology*
(Regency. Zondervan, US. Paternoster Press UK. 1986).

Resources for the church in creation

James Thwaites follows a list of networks that are also engaged in encouraging and equipping those who work in the healthcare sphere.

Healthcare Christian Fellowship International: www.hcfi.info

Nurses Christian Fellowship International: www.ncfi.org

Healthcare in Christ, Australia: www.hcic.org.au

Christian Medical Fellowship, UK: www.cmf.org.uk

International Christian Medical and Dental Association: www.cmda.org

Prime Network, UK: www.prime-international.org.uk

International Hospital Federation: www.ihf-fih.org

teleios resource: theology at work in creation

teleios resource focuses on equipping believers in Christ to engage more fully in their life, work and worship in God's creation. Whilst teleios resource is not an intentional community or movement, it does seek to encourage connections between people of similar interests; particularly in regards to their work in the spheres of creation.

The purpose of teleios resource is to generate opportunities for people to share with and encourage others with the wisdom they are exploring and/or have discovered in their work. Teleios resource also seeks to more fully align the church gathered (as per 1 Tim. 3:15) with the church in all creation (as per Eph. 1:22-23). Also teleios resource engages with individuals, congregations, not-for-profits and for-profit businesses, assisting them, via consultation, mentoring, workshops, conferences and publications.

The key focus of teleios resource is best described by Ephesians 3:9-11, which speaks of *'the administration of the mystery which for ages has been hidden in God who created all things; [this] so that the manifold wisdom of God might now be made known through the church to the rulers and the authorities in the heavenly places... [all this] in accordance with the eternal purpose which [God] carried out in Christ Jesus our Lord'*. Our conviction is that this key text can only be fully understood by placing it within the ancient Hebraic understanding of the creation design and its purpose.

Here follows contacts for those interested in **teleios resource**

The web address of teleios resource is: www.teleios.org.au
Facebook Page: James Thwaites/teleios resource
Email: james.thwaites.77@facebook.com
Teleios Email: teleios_co@bigpond.com

Lightning Source UK Ltd.
Milton Keynes UK
UKOW03f1116221113

221616UK00002B/7/P